The Complementary Therapist's Guide to Red Flags and Referrals

For Elsevier:
Content Strategist: Claire Wilson
Content Development Specialist: Carole McMurray
Project Manager: Srividhya Vidhyashankar
Designer: Miles Hitchen
Illustration Manager: Jennifer Rose

The Complementary Therapist's Guide to Red Flags and Referrals

Clare Stephenson
General Practitioner (GP)
Oxford

Forewords by
Sandy Fritz BS, MS
Owner/Director, Health Enrichment Center Inc., Lapeer MI, USA

Val Hopwood FRCP
Course Director, MSc Acupuncture in Health Care Physiotherapy
& Dietetics, Health and Life Sciences, Coventry University, Coventry, UK

William Morris PhD, DAOM, LAc
President, AOMA Graduate School of Integrative Medicine,
Austin TX, USA

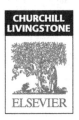

CHURCHILL
LIVINGSTONE

ELSEVIER

EDINBURGH   LONDON   NEW YORK   OXFORD   PHILADELPHIA
ST LOUIS   SYDNEY   TORONTO   2013

CHURCHILL
LIVINGSTONE
ELSEVIER

ISBN: 978-0-7020-4766-4

British Library Cataloguing in Publication Data
A catalogue record for this book is available from the British Library

Library of Congress Cataloging in Publication Data
A catalog record for this book is available from the Library of Congress

Notices
Knowledge and best practice in this field are constantly changing. As new research and experience broaden our understanding, changes in research methods, professional practices, or medical treatment may become necessary.

Practitioners and researchers must always rely on their own experience and knowledge in evaluating and using any information, methods, compounds, or experiments described herein. In using such information or methods they should be mindful of their own safety and the safety of others, including parties for whom they have a professional responsibility.

With respect to any drug or pharmaceutical products identified, readers are advised to check the most current information provided (i) on procedures featured or (ii) by the manufacturer of each product to be administered, to verify the recommended dose or formula, the method and duration of administration, and contraindications. It is the responsibility of practitioners, relying on their own experience and knowledge of their patients, to make diagnoses, to determine dosages and the best treatment for each individual patient, and to take all appropriate safety precautions.

To the fullest extent of the law, neither the Publisher nor the authors, contributors, or editors, assume any liability for any injury and/or damage to persons or property as a matter of products liability, negligence or otherwise, or from any use or operation of any methods, products, instructions, or ideas contained in the material herein.

your source for books,
journals and multimedia
in the health sciences

www.elsevierhealth.com

Printed in China

Contents

Chapter 3
B tables: red flags ordered by symptom keyword   113

Chapter 4
C tables: red flags requiring urgent referral   161

Preface

Over the years in which I have been involved in the training of complementary medical practitioners, I have been struck by how frequently I have been consulted by students and also established therapists who were concerned about their ability to recognise whether or not the clients they were treating had an illness which merited referral for Western medical attention. Despite a rigorous grounding in the basics of clinical medicine and access to good-quality medical textbooks, it is often difficult for a therapist in practice to discern whether the unique symptoms of a particular patient, for example their headaches, their irregular bowel habit or their skin rashes, correlate with those serious conditions which require medical attention. For the practitioner in this position there is inevitably a tension between being safe and being unnecessarily over-concerned.

Medical doctors also have to deal with comparable dilemmas in clinical practice. When can a patient be safely reassured and when do they need further investigation or treatment? To deal with this dilemma, doctors are trained in the recognition of 'red flags'. Red flags are those clinical syndromes which alert the doctor to the fact that the patient needs prompt investigation and treatment for a potentially dangerous condition. Increasingly, doctors have access to excellent guidelines based on expert opinion and clinical research which offer advice on how to respond appropriately to red flags. This means that, ideally, patients are held in a safety net when they explain their symptoms to a doctor. If a red flag, such as the appearance of blood in the sputum, is presented to the doctor, then that patient, like any others who might present to a doctor with a similar pattern of symptoms, will be promptly and appropriately referred for specialist investigations and treatment according to up-to-date guidelines.

It is important for complementary therapists to be aware of these medical red flags. However, in many situations, recognition of medical red flags requires particular medical expertise in examination and interpretation of medical tests. For this reason, there is a clear need for a summary of red flags designed especially for practitioners trained in the professions allied to medicine, such as physiotherapy and nursing, as well as complementary medical therapists. Such a summary should offer guidance on how to respond to those symptoms and signs of disease which can be readily discerned through routine history-taking and basic examination of the body. The guidance needs to be presented in language which does not require full medical training for comprehension. It also needs to offer clear advice on how to respond appropriately when a red flag situation is discerned.

This guide has been written to meet this need. It begins with a definition of red flags as they are presented in the text. Broadly speaking, for the allied and complementary medical therapist, a red flag constitutes any syndrome of symptoms or signs which indicates that the patient might benefit from or require being referred to a doctor *over and above the benefit they could receive from the treatment which might be offered by the therapist.* There are many self-limiting or chronic medical conditions which do not need rapid review by a medical doctor. Conditions such as tension headaches, uncomplicated low back pain, painful periods and irritable bowel syndrome can all be safely treated by non-medically trained therapists. It can be argued that with such functional conditions, the patients are as likely to benefit from treatment from a therapist as they are from seeing a doctor and, more importantly, are very unlikely to come to any harm if a visit to the doctor is delayed by undertaking another form of therapy.

However, if the patient's symptoms or signs indicate that because of the advice, tests or treatment which a doctor is trained to offer, they might benefit from also seeing a doctor for their condition, then it is only right for the allied and complementary therapist to advise the patient to also seek a medical opinion. It is good professional practice to enable the patient to do this in the most efficient way, and making an appropriate referral is part of the process of responding to red flags.

This guide presents tables of red flags in three formats, designed to meet differing needs in training and practice. The first set, the **A tables** (in Chapter 2), order red flags in a systematic way. The **A tables** are ordered according to the physiological systems of the body. This format is intended for the study of red flags, and for understanding how they are outward manifestations of disordered physiological processes in the body. These tables offer some detail about disease processes, but, for an in-depth explanation of how disease might manifest in particular symptoms and signs, the student is urged to consult the sister text to this guide, *The Complementary Therapist's Guide to Conventional Medicine.*[1]

The second set, the **B tables** (in Chapter 3), present red flags according to symptom keyword. These are designed for the practitioner in the clinical situation who is faced with a patient who is presenting with symptoms and signs of a medical condition. These tables are designed to help the practitioner to discern whether or not the symptoms and signs might have any features which suggest serious disease. These tables are cross-referenced to the **A tables** in which more explanation about disease processes can be found.

The final set of tables, the **C tables** (in Chapter 4), present only those relatively few red flags which require a prompt and appropriate response from the practitioner in that urgent referral is merited, and first-aid treatment may be necessary. The reader is advised to commit the red flag conditions of the **C tables** to memory, because in urgent red flag situations there is no time to consult textbooks. These urgent red flag tables will also provide a logical structure around which first-aid training for complementary therapists can be provided.

All the tables indicate with what degree of urgency a therapist needs to respond to red flags. For the large majority of red flags, a non-urgent response is merited.

---

[1]Stephenson C 2011 The Complementary Therapist's Guide to Conventional Medicine. Elsevier, Edinburgh

However, in some cases, a same-day medical assessment or emergency services call out would be best practice, and the reader is offered clear guidance when a rapid response is required.

The book concludes with information on how to make medical referrals, whether this is by letter, by telephone or simply by suggesting the patient makes an appointment to see their doctor. Sample letters are provided so that referral letters can be structured in a way which is familiar to medical doctors and which enables them to gather the crucial information about a case with ease. Appropriately structured referrals have the additional benefit of being a channel of communication with local medical practitioners and can help forge good interprofessional relationships.

The overarching aim of this guide is to improve the confidence, safety and professional integrity of allied and complementary therapists, so that ultimately these qualities will enhance the outcomes of therapeutic encounters with patients.

Clare Stephenson
Oxford
October 2012

Forewords

As a long time massage therapist, instructor and textbook author, I find this text a perfect companion for professional practice. The content is clear, concise and easy to use. Often massage therapy education is not comprehensive enough to assure that the student is competent in making decisions about when a client needs to be referred to a physician. The main reasons for this are the length of many massage training programs and the curriculum content. The student understands the importance of referral but simply does not have adequate time to learn all the specifics. This text solves this problem, not just for the new practitioner but also for those who have been in practice for some time and need a quick reference text.

As an educator, the chapter on how to make a referral is especially important in creating a respectful working relationship among professionals. The differentiation of three categories of red flags is an effective approach in helping the massage therapist as well as other complementary practitioners make appropriate decisions about when a client is in immediate danger and when the condition presents as non-urgent but will need referral for follow-up.

I also believe that this text will help physicians feel more confident about including massage and other complementary therapies in the comprehensive treatment plan for their patients because the information clearly indicates when and how to refer, and opens dialogue for the best care of the clients/patients. It is important that all health care professionals have the information necessary to work together for the good of the client/patient. Information to support clinical decision making is essential. The information in this text allows the practitioner to provide services in a safe manner because they are aware of the red flags. I am thankful to the author for considering the inclusion of complementary health care therapists into current health care systems and creating a reference to make the path of integrated health practice smoother.

Sandy Fritz BS, MS
Owner/Director
Health Enrichment Center Inc.
Lapeer MI, USA (2012)

Using any kind of medicine is a chancy business but complementary medicine is thought to be generally benign. However, any practitioner, if they are honest, will tell you of patients where they have had doubts, sudden sinking feelings or nagging little puzzles about the safety and advisability of treatment when dealing with a patient even though they may have a clear Western diagnosis. Those of us trained in Western medicine expect to feel secure in our abilities but often complementary therapy takes us out of our comfort zone.

This book answers a long unarticulated need. An authoritative guide to the theory and use of the red flag system is almost as good as having a wise advisor by your shoulder in clinic. It means that we can concentrate on helping the patient recover with less anxiety that we might somehow be making their condition worse.

The logical arrangement of the text is really helpful and designed to prioritise the information in a very practical way. While it would be ideal to have plenty of time to sit down and think about all the issues, this book will allow a hasty consultation and guide the reader to the relative urgency of the most important symptoms quickly. The distinction between "high priority" and "urgent" is helpful to consider. That the summary tables, A and B, are presented in different ways is an innovative design, allowing for those who think first in physiological terms to integrate with those who may focus primarily on organ systems (TCM practitioners). Even more important for quick reference is the inclusion of first aid suggestions in the C group of tables. The section on communicating with medical practitioners is brief and vital for sensible inter-professional communication at any time.

To sum up, this is a book I would have been very grateful for as a student physiotherapist and will still find invaluable as a practising acupuncturist. Dr Stephenson has gently inserted an extra layer of protection for all our patients.

Val Hopwood FRCP
Course Director
MSc Acupuncture in Health
Care Physiotherapy & Dietetics
Health and Life Sciences, Coventry University
Coventry, UK (2012)

Red Flags and Referrals addresses a need throughout the educational systems of Integrative and Complementary and Alternative Medicine (CAM) practices. The process of collaboration is one of communication, and the skills addressed in this text provide the necessary tools for professional referral in the sense of best practices.

CAM practices are some of the safest. The agents used are generally of low toxicity and there are few if any adverse events reported in a given year[1].

Take acupuncture, for instance. Ernst et al. reviewed data collected over a ten-year period, listing 165 references, 32 of which were systematic reviews[2]. They identified 38 cases of infection, 42 traumas, 13 adverse effects and five deaths, many of which had tenuous claims relating them to acupuncture.

By comparison, the 1994 report on adverse drug reactions by Lazarou et al. analyzed 33 million US hospital admissions. They concluded that prescription drugs caused 2.2 million serious injuries. Further, fatal adverse drug reactions occurred in 0.19% of in-patients and 0.13% of admissions. They projected that 106,000 deaths occur annually due to adverse drug reactions[3].

This comparison between risks related to CAM practices and conventional practices is highlighted here for one reason. This risk for CAM is not in the products, rather it is in the knowledge and skill of the practitioner in terms of appropriate and ethical referrals. There have been no texts that fulfil this knowledge area for the CAM provider until now. This book fills that gap and does an excellent job.

The risk in the CAM provider resides within the ability to identify red flags, thereby making timely and appropriate referrals. Critical features of the process are addressed, such as prioritizing red flags in terms of non-urgent, high priority and urgent.

William Morris PhD, DAOM, LAc
President
AOMA Graduate School of Integrative Medicine
Austin TX, USA (2012)

REFERENCES

1. Rogers, P., 1998. Serious Complications of Acupuncture … Or Acupuncture Abuses? (An edited version of the original in the American Journal of Acupuncture Oct–Dec 1981: 9(4); 347–351).

2. Ernst, E., Myeong, S.L., Choi, T.Y., 2011. Acupuncture: Does it alleviate pain and are there serious risks? A review of reviews. PAIN® 152 (4).

3. Lazarou, J., Pomeranz, B.H., Corey, P.N., 1998. Incidence of Adverse Drug Reactions in Hospitalized Patients. JAMA: The Journal of the American Medical Association 279 (15), 1200–1205.

Acknowledgements

The creation of this book was inspired by my contact with successive
"generations" of students of acupuncture at the College of Integrated Chinese
Medicine in Reading, UK. Over the years of teaching these students, this guide
to Red Flags and Referrals evolved in response to their expressed need for
confidence when dealing with patients with potentially worrying symptoms and
signs. Moreover, this guide was very much shaped by the feedback these students
gave to the emerging text. It has been very inspiring to witness that for so many
of these individuals, now mature practitioners, their commitment continues to be
to offer to their patients treatment which is holistic in the best possible sense of
the word and in which safety is paramount. This text is dedicated to these
students, now practitioners, and also to all complementary therapists whose
primary aim as practitioners is to make the treatment room a safe place of healing
for their patients. As a practising GP I am indebted to those therapists who work
close to me, to whom I know I can refer my patients in the confidence that they
will receive highly supportive care and very safe treatment.

I also have much gratitude to Angela and John Hicks and Peter Mole,
the founders of the College of Integrated Chinese Medicine, who continue to
teach and inspire students at the college. From the outset they supported my
enthusiasm to develop teaching materials about conventional medicine for their
students. They then very generously encouraged me to submit these materials
written for the college as material to be considered for publication. Without their
support this and the sister text, *The Complementary Therapist's Guide to Clinical
Medicine,* could not have been published.

I must also extend many thanks to Claire Wilson, Carole McMurray and
Srividhya Vidhyashankar from Elsevier who have seen the original text through
the process of development into a form which can be used as a handy reference in
the treatment room.

Finally, my thanks have to go to John Wheeler who has over the course of four
years patiently encouraged me in the transformation of the teaching materials into
copy for a textbook, and also edited and proofread much of the text. Without
him I could never have produced this completed version.

CHAPTER 1

RED FLAGS OF DISEASE

Red flags are those symptoms and signs which, if elicited by therapist, either of conventional or complementary medicine, merit referral to a conventional doctor. Referral is indicated because the presence of red flags indicates the possibility of a condition which either may not respond fully to non-medical treatment or may benefit further from conventional diagnosis, advice or treatment.

In summary, referral may be considered for the following four broad reasons:

1. To enable the patient to have access to medical treatment which will benefit their condition.
2. For investigations to exclude the possibility of serious disease.
3. For investigations to confirm a diagnosis and help guide treatment.
4. For access to advice on the management of a complex condition.

It is important to clarify at this stage that the red flags indicate those potentially serious conditions in which the patient would be in need of further tests, advice or treatment. Not all of the red flag conditions listed in this text indicate that the patient will need medical treatment. In some cases referral is advised so that the patient can have tests to exclude an unlikely but important treatable condition (e.g. a mole that might have features of skin cancer), or to obtain a medical diagnosis to guide in the future management of the condition (e.g. ascertaining the severity and cause of suspected anaemia). In other situations it may be important to refer so that the patient can have access to detailed medical advice (e.g. on the complexity of assessing coronary risk and how this impacts on subsequent choice of medical treatment).

USE OF COMPLEMENTARY MEDICINE AND RED FLAGS

There are very few examples of when complementary medicine would not be beneficial to someone who is also receiving conventional investigation or treatment for a condition. Therefore, referral in response of a patient with red flag symptoms or signs does not mean that complementary medical treatment need be discontinued, as long as the therapist is sure that the patient has given informed consent to this treatment.

THE RED FLAGS AS GUIDES TO REFERRAL

Red flags are guides to referral and not absolute indicators. Often the red flags described in this text specify a fixed, measurable point at which referral should be

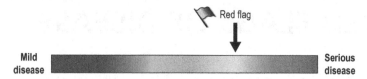

These red flags are guides for referral and not absolute indicators of serious disease

Figure 1.1 This illustrates the fact that red flags have to fall at a fixed point along the spectrum of symptoms of mild to serious disease.

considered, for example high fever (especially if over 40°C) not responding to treatment within 2 hours in a child. Of course, in reality, disease falls somewhere along a spectrum which bridges the state of being of little concern and one of being of serious concern (see Figure 1.1). A disease does not suddenly become serious once a fixed point has passed. Moreover, what might constitute a red flag in one individual may be of less concern in someone of a stronger constitution.

Bearing the potential flexibility of interpretation of red flag syndromes in mind, there may well be situations in which the clinical opinion of the therapist is that referral is unnecessary even though a red flag is present. Conversely if a nagging uncertainty persists in a clinical situation, even if the patient does not fit the criteria for any of the red flags, then it is safest to trust clinical instincts and refer. The important thing is that there is an awareness of these indicators of possible serious disease, and that in every case time has been taken to consider their relevance for patients in the clinical situation.

PRIORITISATION OF THE RED FLAGS

The various red flags merit different responses from the practitioner according to the nature of the underlying condition of which they may be an indication. To aid with decision making in the clinical situation, the red flags listed in this text are assigned to one or more of three categories of urgency.

These categories are:

*Non-urgent: A non-urgent referral means that the patient can be encouraged to make a routine appointment with the medical practitioner (GP) and this ideally will take place within 7 days at the most.
**High priority: A high priority referral means that the patient is assessed by a medical practitioner within the same day.
***Urgent: The urgent category is for those situations when the patient requires immediate medical attention, and this may mean summoning an on-call doctor or calling the paramedics to the scene.

The summaries of red flags which make up the appendix to this chapter indicate which category (ies) of urgency best fits each red flag. Again, this categorisation is simply a guide to the degree of urgency rather than a fixed directive on the appropriate response in a particular clinical situation.

For many of the listed red flags, the labelling indicates a range of degrees of priority (for example, */**). For these red flags, the precise level of priority depends upon other characteristics of the individual case, which should become clear according to the particular clinical situation.

HOW TO RESPOND TO THE RED FLAGS

The response to a red flag in a clinical situation depends very much upon what degree of urgency the response merits. In this book, the detail of the advice given relates to the practicalities of referral to a GP or emergency hospital department within the UK National Health Service. However, this advice is readily transferable to any national provider of medical health care, as in all there are systems whereby a generalist doctor can be consulted for non-urgent medical conditions and emergency services can be accessed for conditions requiring urgent medical assessment.

NON-URGENT RED FLAGS

Some red flags are indicators of possible serious disease, and yet the patient does not require urgent treatment, even if the disease actually is present. An example of this is the patient who has features of anaemia, including pallor, breathlessness and palpitations on exertion. Anaemia can have serious underlying causes, for example chronic gastrointestinal bleeding or pernicious anaemia, some of which cannot be expected to respond fully to non-medical therapies. In a case of anaemia, the patient obviously requires further investigation and may possibly require medical treatment according to the outcome of the investigations. However, if the symptoms have been developing over the course of weeks to months, the patient does not need to be seen by the doctor on the same day.

Another example of a non-urgent red flag is the well child who has symptoms which indicate occasional bouts of mild asthma. In this case referral is recommended more for confirmation of diagnosis, and so that the patient can have access to medical advice about how to manage a potentially serious condition, rather than simply for treatment. It will be obvious that in such a situation the child does not need to be seen urgently.

Most of the red flags of cancer have been prioritised as of non-urgent priority. This is because such features usually have taken weeks to develop, and 1 or 2 days' delay is not critical in the course of most cancers. In the UK, the NHS referral system is structured so that the patient demonstrating red flag signs of cancer is seen by a hospital specialist within 2 weeks of referral by their GP, so to be seen by the GP within only a few days of referral would be ideal in order to minimise the total wait. Of course, there will be some situations in which it would be appropriate to make a high priority referral for patients showing features of cancer, either because of rapidity of progression of symptoms, or in order to allay anxiety for the patient.

Those red flags which have been categorised as non-urgent will require non-urgent referral. In these situations it can be suggested to the patient to make a non-urgent appointment with the GP. This means that the patient will be seen within the next few days. In this situation a letter of referral can be prepared, although this may not be necessary if the patient is capable of passing on the essential information verbally. If a letter is needed, it can either be taken to the doctor by the patient (most reliable approach) or can be sent by post to the practice (more likely to be delayed or go astray). A guide to writing letters of referral to doctors can be found in Chapter 5, 'Communicating with medical professionals'.

HIGH PRIORITY RED FLAGS

Some of the listed red flags are indicators of serious disease, and these merit seeking a medical opinion on the same day, because there is a possibility that the condition of the patient might deteriorate rapidly without treatment. An example of a high priority case is the situation of haemoptysis (coughing up blood) in a man who has lost two stone in weight over the past few months (strong indicators of lung cancer or TB). In this case, the potential of serious blood loss or the possibility of contagiousness makes the referral high priority.

In high priority situations, it may be best practice to speak to the patient's medical doctor. It is appropriate in such cases to telephone the patient's practice to confirm a time in that day when it is most convenient to talk to one of the doctors. After discussion, if the doctor agrees with your assessment of urgency, an appropriate appointment for the patient can be made.

Alternatively, it may be more appropriate that patients make these referrals themselves, and they can be advised to request a same day appointment with their doctor.

In such situations it is good practice to give the patient a letter describing the clinical findings and concerns to take to their doctor before they leave your clinic. In a high priority case, a hand-written referral letter on headed note-paper is acceptable (see also Chapter 5).

URGENT RED FLAGS

In some cases the red flags indicate that the patient requires urgent medical assessment. In these cases it may be appropriate to request an emergency ambulance to take the patient to hospital. A less dramatic option is to telephone the patient's practice to ask to speak to a doctor urgently in order to get their advice about referral to hospital. If there is some uncertainty, the doctor may choose to visit the patient first, or ask for them to come to the practice to be seen before the paramedics are called.

In those urgent cases in which it is unlikely that the therapist will meet the examining doctor, it is good practice to hand-write the reason for referral in a letter which is either to be taken with the patient to the hospital or to be given to the doctor when they arrive.

THE SUMMARIES OF RED FLAGS OF DISEASE

The red flags of disease are summarised in Chapters 2, 3 and 4. Each table presents information about red flags in a different way to meet the needs presented by different clinical situations. In the **A tables** (Chapter 2), red flags are presented according to the physiological system of the body in which the disease they indicate might have become manifest. This is the way in which information is ordered within a medical textbook. If the red flags are to be incorporated into a structured teaching programme on clinical medicine, this structure enables the red flags to be taught in a systematic way. This part of the guide also gives some explanation as to why the red flag syndromes merit consideration for referral.

However, in the clinic situation, symptoms do not arise in a systematic way. Rather, in the clinic the question 'Is this symptom/sign serious?' is more likely to be asked than 'I wonder if there are any serious symptoms arising from this patient's digestive system?' The **B tables** (Chapter 3) present the red flags according to symptom keyword (e.g. headache, abdominal pain, eye problem, menstrual disorder) to enable easy reference in a clinical situation. The **B tables** give less detailed explanatory information, but each red flag listed is referenced to the more detailed summary given in the **A tables** so that more information can quickly be found if needed.

Finally, the list of red flags has been further pared down in the **C tables** (Chapter 4) to a summary of urgent red flags which summarise those high priority and urgent situations in which first-aid management is indicated. These tables also give some guidance on first-aid treatments. This guidance is intended to supplement the regular first-aid training which all complementary medical practitioners are required to undergo. These are the red flags that it is worth taking time to understand and to commit to memory in order to be fully prepared to act appropriately should a situation of medical urgency arise in the clinic.

CHAPTER 2

A TABLES: RED FLAGS ORDERED BY PHYSIOLOGICAL SYSTEM

INTRODUCTION

These A tables are ordered according to the physiological systems of the body. Each A table lists the red flags which are related to disease of that physiological system. The red flags are defined according to symptoms (the patient's experience of disease) and/or signs (measurable physiological changes of disease). These tables also offer a brief explanation as to why the constellation of symptoms and signs constitute a red flag. These tables are introduced and explained in more depth in the relevant chapters of the companion text *The Complementary Therapist's Guide to Clinical Medicine* to which the readers are referred should they wish to study these patterns of disease in more depth.

The A tables show the categorisation of urgency of referral which is described in Chapter 1:

*Non-urgent: a non-urgent referral means that the patient can be encouraged to make a routine appointment with the medical practitioner (GP) and this ideally will take place within 7 days at the most.

**High priority: a high priority referral means that the patient is assessed by a medical practitioner within the same day. This can be either as a home visit or at the medical practice.

***Urgent: the urgent category is for those situations when the patient requires immediate medical attention, and this may mean summoning an on-call doctor or calling the paramedics to the scene.

The order of the A tables can be found in the contents pages of this text.

A1: RED FLAGS OF CANCER

Cancer is characterized by progressive growth of diseased tissue over the course of weeks to months and the loss of function which can result from the damage caused by this growth. The patient may therefore experience a deterioration in function which may either be gradual or may appear with the sudden development of new symptoms which do not go away. The red flags of cancer include any progressive unexplained symptoms which persist over the course of weeks to months without resolution. Also unexplained sizeable lumps and lymph nodes may be indicative of cancerous change.

TABLE A1 Red flags of cancer

Red flag	Description	Reasoning	Priority
A1.1	**Progressive unexplained symptoms** over weeks to months: e.g. **weight loss**, **recurrent sweats** (especially at night), **fevers** and **poor appetite**	Symptoms that progress (i.e. gradually worsen rather than fluctuate in intensity) over this sort of time period are strongly suggestive of cancer NB: There is usually no need to request a high priority referral when wanting to exclude a diagnosis of cancer, as this might increase rather than allay anxiety. Only consider high priority referral if you suspect rapidly progressive disease, or if the patient is already very anxious	**/*
A1.2	**An unexplained lump >1 cm in diameter:** characteristically **hard**, **irregular**, **fixed** and **painless**	Cancerous lumps are usually irregular, may be fixed to associated tissues, and often are painless unless they obstruct viscera, cause pressure on other structures, grow into bone or grow into nerve roots Soft round mobile lumps are more likely to be benign tumours. Painful lumps are more characteristic of inflammation or infection than cancer	**/*
A1.3	**Unexplained bleeding:** either from the surface of the skin, or emerging from an internal organ such as the bowel, bladder or uterus (e.g. **blood in vomit**, **blood in urine**, **rectal bleeding** or **vaginal bleeding**)	Cancerous tissue is poorly organised, and bleeding may easily be provoked from the surface of an epithelial tumour (e.g. of breast, skin, lung, mouth, stomach, bowel, bladder or uterus)	**/*

TABLE A1 Continued

Red flag	Description	Reasoning	Priority
A1.4	**Features of bone marrow failure:** severe progressive **anaemia** (see **A18.2**), recurrent progressive **infections** or **bruising**, **purpura** and **bleeding**	Secondary cancer and cancer of the blood cells often infiltrate the bone marrow and prevent it from performing its role of producing healthy red and white blood cells and platelets Purpura is pin-point bruising, which looks like a rash of flat, purplish spots, and is one of the signs of a low platelet count (see also **A20.1**)	***/**
A1.5	**Multiple enlarged lymph nodes** (>1 cm in diameter), painless, with no other obvious cause (e.g. known glandular fever infection) and lasting for more than 2 weeks	Groups of lymph nodes can be found in the cervical region, in the armpits (axillary nodes) and in the inguinal creases (groin). In health, lymph nodes are usually soft, impalpable masses of soft tissue, but these can enlarge and become more palpable when the node is active in fighting an infection, or if it is infiltrated by tumour cells. If a number of nodes are enlarged (to >1 cm in diameter), this may signify a generalised infectious disease such as glandular fever or human immunodeficiency virus (HIV) infection The other important cause of widespread lymph node enlargement (lymphadenopathy) is disseminated cancer, in particular the cancers of the white blood cells (leukaemia and lymphoma) If multiple enlarged lymph nodes are found it is best to refer for a diagnosis, and as a high priority if the patient is unwell with other symptoms	**/*
A1.6	**A single, markedly enlarged lymph node** (>2 cm in diameter) with no other obvious cause	Even in the situation of infection it is unusual for a lymph node to become very enlarged. Cancerous infiltration can lead to a firm enlarged lymph node which may be painless. This is particularly typical of lymphoma	**/*

TABLE A1 Continued

Red flag	Description	Reasoning	Priority
A1.7	**Painless abdominal swelling or bloating** due to fluid accumulation (ascites)	Abdominal epithelial malignancies such as colon cancer, stomach cancer and ovarian cancer may lead to the accumulation of fluid within the abdominal cavity, which initially may be painless. This sign is known as 'ascites'. Ascites is a sign that the cancer has metastasised, and so carries a poor prognosis. Other causes of ascites include chronic congestive cardiac failure, liver failure and kidney disease Bloating after meals or at the end of the day is not usually a serious sign, and more commonly is a feature of irritable bowel syndrome. However, progressive abdominal bloating over the course of weeks may indicate tumour bulk (particularly in ovarian cancer), and merits referral	

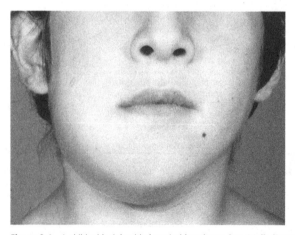

Figure 2.1 A child with right-sided cervical lymphoma (see A1.6). (From Kumar and Clark, 6th edn, Figure 9.14.)

A2: RED FLAGS OF INFECTIOUS DISEASES: VULNERABLE GROUPS

Infections are more likely to cause problems in individuals who cannot sustain a strong immune response, either because of immaturity, old age, illness, pregnancy or because of exposure to unusual organisms (such as occurs during foreign travel).

TABLE A2 Red flags of infectious diseases: vulnerable groups

Red flag	Description	Reasoning	Priority
Treat anyone from the following vulnerable groups with caution if they are displaying features of an infectious disease (e.g. **fever**, **confusion**, **diarrhoea** and **vomiting**, **spreading areas** of **inflammation** or **yellowish discharges**)			
A2.1	**Infants** (especially if <3 months old)	Infections in infants can become serious conditions very quickly because of the immature immune system, poor temperature control and small size. They lead easily to high fever and dehydration The infant is at increased risk of convulsions and circulatory collapse However, in this age group fever is common, and usually is *not* serious	**
A2.2	The **elderly**	Infections can take hold rapidly in the elderly because of a weakened immune system. Serious disease can 'hide' behind mild-appearing symptoms	**
A2.3	The **immunocompromised**	The immunocompromised are particularly vulnerable to severe overwhelming infections, in particular of the respiratory and gastrointestinal systems	**
A2.4	In **pregnancy**	Certain infections can directly damage the embryo/fetus or lead to miscarriage. Others may be transmitted to the baby during labour Prolonged high fever may induce miscarriage or early labour	**
A2.5	Anyone with a **recent history of travel** to a tropical country (within the past month)	Certain tropical diseases (including malaria) can become rapidly overwhelming and may present up to 4 weeks after return from the tropical country	**

A3: RED FLAGS OF INFECTIOUS DISEASES: FEVER, DEHYDRATION AND CONFUSION

Fever can be assessed by means of thermometers of various designs which may measure body temperature from various locations in the body (e.g. forehead skin, ear, rectum and mouth). The measured temperature is slightly different according to the site, so it is important to be clear from the thermometer manufacturer's instructions what the normal range is for the device which is being used.

The core temperature of a well person tends to follow a diurnal variation with core temperature peaking in the late afternoon at up to 1°C (1.8F) higher than the temperature measured in the early morning. Also, for temperatures less then 37.5°C (99.5F) what is normal for one person may represent a fever in another who tends to run at a generally lower core temperature. This makes interpretation of lower levels of fever difficult, and in such cases it is very helpful to know what the normal range is for that person in health.

Increasingly the tympanic (eardrum) temperature is rapidly assessed by means of user-friendly hand-held devices. The normal ranges below represent tympanic readings in adults. The tympanic temperature range is higher than the oral range by up to 0.7°C, and so the guidance below should be adjusted accordingly if oral readings are being interpreted. It must also be remembered that the normal range of temperature for children is slightly higher than for adults (see below).

TABLE A3 Red flags of infectious diseases: fever, dehydration and confusion

Red flag	Description	Reasoning	Priority
Definitions: *Normal body (tympanic) temperature:* 36.8 ± 0.7°C (98.2F ± 1.3F) 37.5°C is the upper limit of normal for teenagers and adults *Fever:* body temperature >37.5°C (99.5F) *Moderate fever:* 37.5–38.5°C (99.5–101.3F) *High fever:* body temperature >38.5°C (>101.3F) 38.0°C (100.4F) is the upper limit of normal tympanic temperature for infants (up to 2 years) 37.8°C (100F) is the upper limit of normal for older children (between 3–10 years of age)			
A3.1	**High fever in a child** (<8 years old) not responding to treatment within 2 hours	High fevers can promote infantile convulsions in young children. Treatment to bring the temperature down includes keeping the environment cool, tepid sponging and approaches such as acupuncture or homeopathy. Antipyretic medication such as paracetamol or ibuprofen suspension could be considered	**

TABLE A3 Continued

Red flag	Description	Reasoning	Priority
A3.2	**High fever in an older child or adult** that does not respond to treatment within 48 hours	Although risk of convulsions is low in this group of patients, a high fever is very depleting and can lead to dehydration. If a high fever is not responding to your treatment in 2 days, this suggests the possibility of a serious condition which merits further investigations	**
A3.3	**Any fever** of unknown cause that persists for or recurs over >2 weeks	Most mild infectious diseases have run their course within a week; a prolonged fever suggests either a chronic inflammatory or infectious condition, or cancer, all of which merit further investigations	**/*
A3.4	**Dehydration in an infant:** signs include dry mouth and skin, loss of skin turgor (firmness), drowsiness, sunken fontanelle and dry nappies	A dehydrated infant is at high risk of circulatory collapse because of its small size and immature homeostatic mechanisms. Infants who are dehydrated may lose the desire to drink, and so the condition can rapidly deteriorate	***/**
A3.5	**Dehydration in older children and adults** if severe or prolonged for >48 hours. Signs include: dry mouth and skin, loss of skin turgor, low blood pressure, dizziness on standing and poor urine output	Although not as unstable as an infant, a dehydrated child or adult still needs hydration to prevent damage to the kidneys. Referral should be made if the patient is unable to take fluids or if the dehydration persists for >48 hours. Refer elderly people immediately, as the ability to take in fluids is often reduced and the kidneys and brain are more vulnerable to damage	**
A3.6	**Confusion in older children and adults with fever**	Confusion is common and benign in young children (<8 years of age) and elderly frail people when a fever develops. However, it is not usual in healthy adults, and should be referred to exclude central nervous system involvement (e.g. meningitis, brain abscess). Refer in all cases if the confusion might pose a risk to the patient or to others	**
A3.7	**Febrile convulsion in child:** ongoing	Refer a case in which the convulsion is not settling within 2 minutes as an emergency. Ensure the child is kept in a safe place and in the recovery position while help arrives	***

TABLE A3 Continued

Red flag	Description	Reasoning	Priority
A3.8	**Febrile convulsion in child:** recovered	Refer all cases in which the child has just suffered a febrile convulsion (the parents need advice on how to manage future fits, and the child should be examined by a doctor)	**

A4: RED FLAGS OF DISEASES OF THE MOUTH

TABLE A4 Red flags of diseases of the mouth

Red flag	Description	Reasoning	Priority
A4.1	**Persistent oral thrush (candidiasis)** (appearing as a thick white coating on tongue or palate)	Although common in the newborn, oral thrush in children and adults is not a normal finding, and merits referral to exclude an underlying cause. Common causes include corticosteroid use (including asthma inhalers), diabetes, immunodeficiency (including HIV/AIDS) and cancer. Dentures in elderly people can also predispose to oral thrush	*
A4.2	**Persistent painless white plaque (leukoplakia)** (appearing as a coating that appears to sit on the surface of the sides of the tongue)	Leukoplakia is a pre-cancerous change that signifies an increased risk of mouth cancer. It is more common in smokers and in those with a high alcohol intake. A particular form of leukoplakia is also associated with HIV/AIDS Early treatment of leukoplakia can prevent invasive mouth cancer, so referral is merited	*
A4.3	**Painless enlargement of a salivary gland** over weeks to months	This needs referral to exclude salivary gland cancer, which is most common in people >60 years old	*
A4.4	**Painful or painless enlargement of salivary gland** immediately after eating	This suggests a salivary gland stone or obstruction from dried secretions. Early treatment is to maximise hydration by encouraging drinking, and to encourage salivation (e.g. with lemon juice). If the problem is persistent, referral is recommended, as surgical removal of the stone may be necessary	*

TABLE A4 Continued

Red flag	Description	Reasoning	Priority
A4.5	**Tender or inflamed gums or salivary glands** which do not respond within days to your treatment	May be accompanied by fever or malaise. These symptoms suggest dental abscess or infection of the salivary gland, and if they persist indicate a need for referral for antibiotic treatment to prevent inflammatory damage to dental roots or salivary glands	**
A4.6	**Ulceration of mouth** if persistent (>1 week) or if preventing proper hydration	The most common cause of painful ulceration of the mouth is herpes simplex virus infection. This can be so severe as to inhibit drinking in a child. If this is the case, the child may need to be hospitalised for rehydration If ulceration persists for >2 weeks it might suggest an underlying inflammatory condition (e.g. Crohn's disease) or mouth cancer, which will require further investigation Rarely, severe mouth ulceration can be the first sign of bone marrow failure (see **A1**), and in this case results from a very low white blood cell count	**

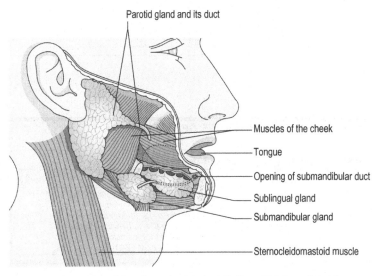

Parotid gland and its duct

Muscles of the cheek

Tongue

Opening of submandibular duct

Sublingual gland

Submandibular gland

Sternocleidomastoid muscle

Figure 2.2 The position of the salivary glands (see A4.3). (From CTG Figure 3.1a-IV.)

A5: RED FLAGS OF DISEASES OF THE OESOPHAGUS

TABLE A5 Red flags of diseases of the oesophagus

Red flag	Description	Reasoning	Priority
A5.1	**Difficulty swallowing (dysphagia), which is worse with solids** (in particular if progressive over days to weeks)	A sensation of difficulty in swallowing or a lump in the throat is a common and often benign symptom, which may fluctuate with emotional stress (a syndrome known as 'globus pharyngeus'). Usually, swallowing of food is still possible with this form of dysphagia However, if there is a physical obstruction in the oesophagus, which may be the result of cancer or stricture (scarring), there may be progressive difficulty in swallowing stiff foods, and this will be accompanied by a loss of weight. This needs prompt referral	**/*
A5.2	**Difficulty swallowing (dysphagia) associated with enlarged lymph nodes in the neck**	(See **A5.1**.) Dysphagia that is also associated with enlarged lymph nodes raises the possibility of a malignant or inflammatory cause, and merits referral	**/*
A5.3	**Swallowing associated with central chest pain** (behind the sternum)	Swallowing that is associated with a delayed pain behind the sternum suggests oesophagitis or structural damage to the oesophagus (e.g. a tear or puncture by a fishbone). Refer if symptoms are not settling within 24 hours, or sooner if pain is severe	*

A6: RED FLAGS OF DISEASES OF THE STOMACH

TABLE A6 Red flags of diseases of the stomach

Red flag	Description	Reasoning	Priority
A6.1	**Severe diarrhoea and vomiting** if lasting >24 hours in infants or the elderly	In most cases diarrhoea and vomiting are self-limiting and will need no medical intervention. However, infants and the elderly are vulnerable to dehydration and should be referred for assessment if symptoms continue for >24 hours	***/**

TABLE A6 Continued

Red flag	Description	Reasoning	Priority
A6.2	**Diarrhoea and vomiting** if continuing for >5 days in otherwise healthy adults	(See **A6.1**.) If symptoms persist for >5 days, this is unusual and merits referral for investigation of infectious or inflammatory causes Food poisoning (diarrhoea and vomiting from contaminated food) and infectious bloody diarrhoea are notifiable diseases.[1] If a notifiable disease is a possibility, the patient should be advised to consult their doctor so that the disease can be reported for the benefit of the public health	**
A6.3	**Diarrhoea and vomiting** associated with features of dehydration (see **A3** – infectious diseases: fever, dehydration and confusion)	If features of dehydration (low blood pressure, dry mouth, concentrated urine, poor skin turgor, confusion) are apparent, refer as a matter of high priority, and urgently in infants and the elderly. In these cases, continuing vomiting will exacerbate an already unstable situation Food poisoning and infectious bloody diarrhoea are notifiable diseases (see **A6.2**)[1]	***/**
A6.4	**Vomiting of fresh blood or altered blood** (looks like dark gravel or coffee grounds)	The appearance of blood in the vomit is always of concern as it is not possible to gauge the severity of bleeding and whether or not the internal bleeding is continuing Refer if more than about a tablespoon of blood appears in the vomit (small amounts may simply be the result of a tear of the oesophagus lining during vomiting) The blood may originate from the stomach or the duodenum and may indicate peptic ulcer disease or stomach cancer Refer urgently if there are any signs of shock (see **A19.3**). Signs of shock indicate that there could be dangerous levels of internal blood loss.	***/**

TABLE A6 Continued

Red flag	Description	Reasoning	Priority
A6.5	**Projectile vomiting** persisting for >2 days	Projectile vomiting (vomit appears at a much higher speed than usual) suggests high obstruction to the outflow of the stomach, and should be referred as there is high risk of loss of fluids and salts Refer as a high priority if this is suspected in a newborn baby (a sign of the congenital deformity of pyloric stenosis)	***/**
A6.6	**Epigastric pain or dyspepsia** for the first time in someone over the age of 40 years or in anyone if resistant to treatment after 6 weeks	Pain from the stomach or duodenum typically radiates to the epigastric region. If the stomach is inflamed, this area can be tender on palpation, and there may be a sensation of acidity or fullness (dyspepsia). However, these symptoms are very common and can respond well to dietary modification and complementary medicine. Only refer if not responding to your treatment within 6 weeks or if presenting for the first time in someone over 40 years old (as the risk of cancer is more common in older age groups) Persistent dyspeptic symptoms may result from *Helicobacter pylori* infection, and may respond well to antibiotic eradication treatment. Chronic *Helicobacter* infection is associated with an increased risk of stomach cancer as well as peptic ulceration, so it is good medical practice for this infection to be treated	*
A6.7	**Altered blood in stools** (melaena): stools look like black tar	Altered blood in stools (stools look tarry and have an unusual metallic smell) indicates bleeding from the more proximal aspects of the digestive tract, including the stomach. If melaena is apparent in the stools then bleeding is significant and merits prompt referral	***/**

TABLE A6 Continued

Red flag	Description	Reasoning	Priority
A6.8	**Onset of severe abdominal pain with collapse** (the acute abdomen): the pain can be constant or colicky (coming in waves); rigidity, guarding and rebound tenderness are serious signs	The 'acute abdomen' is a term that refers to the combination of severe abdominal pain together with an inability to continue with day-to-day activities ('collapse'). This syndrome can have benign causes, such as irritable bowel syndrome, dysmenorrhoea and ovulation pain, but needs high priority or urgent referral to exclude more serious conditions including appendicitis, perforated ulcer, peritonitis, obstructed bowel, pelvic inflammatory disease and gallstones Colicky pain indicates obstruction of a viscus (hollow organ) Rigidity of the abdomen, guarding (a reflex protective spasm of the abdominal muscles) and rebound tenderness (pain felt elsewhere in the abdomen when the pressure of the palpating hand is released) all suggest inflammation or perforation of a viscus	***/**

[1]Notifiable diseases: notification of a number of specified infectious diseases is required of doctors in the UK as a statutory duty under the Public Health (Infectious Diseases) 1988 Act and the Public Health (Control of Diseases) 1988 Act and, more recently, the Health Protection (Notification) Regulations 2010. The UK Health Protection Agency (HPA) Centre for Infections collates details of each case of each disease that has been notified. This allows analyses of local and national trends. This is one example of a situation in which there is a legal requirement for a doctor to breach patient confidentiality.

Diseases that are notifiable include: acute encephalitis, acute poliomyelitis, acute infectious hepatitis, anthrax, cholera, diphtheria, enteric fevers (typhoid and paratyphoid), food poisoning, infectious bloody diarrhoea, leprosy, malaria, measles, meningitis (bacterial and viral forms), meningococcal septicaemia (without meningitis), mumps, plague, rabies, rubella, SARS, scarlet fever, smallpox, tetanus, tuberculosis, typhus, viral haemorrhagic fever, whooping cough and yellow fever.

A7: RED FLAGS OF DISEASES OF THE PANCREAS

TABLE A7 Red flags of diseases of the pancreas

Red flag	Description	Reasoning	Priority
A7.1	**Symptoms of acute pancreatitis:** acute pancreatitis presents as the acute abdomen (see **A6.8**) with severe central abdominal and back pain, vomiting and dehydration	Pancreatitis is a serious inflammatory condition of the pancreas which may develop for no obvious reason, but can be associated with high alcohol consumption or gallstone obstruction. The patient needs to be nil by mouth and urgently referred for supportive hospital care	***
A7.2	**Symptoms of chronic pancreatitis:** central abdominal and back pain, weight loss and loose stools over weeks to months	Chronic pancreatitis may result from long-term alcohol abuse, episodes of acute pancreatitis or be due to inherited tendency. The scarred pancreas can generate deep chronic pain, and the lack of digestive enzymes can lead to the syndrome of malabsorption (see **A7.3**). There is a risk of diabetes	**/*
A7.3	**Malabsorption syndrome:** loose pale stools and malnutrition; weight loss, thin hair, dry skin, cracked lips and peeled tongue Will present as failure to thrive in children	The malabsorption syndrome develops when there is an inability to absorb the nutrients in the diet, and weight loss and mineral and vitamin deficiencies result. Loose stools are the result of the presence of unabsorbed fat Chronic pancreatitis is one of the causes of the malabsorption syndrome (see **A7.2**). Other causes include coeliac disease, Crohn's disease and intestinal lymphoma	**/*
A7.4	**Jaundice:** yellowish skin, yellow whites of the eyes, and possibly dark urine and pale stools; itch may be a prominent symptom	Jaundice results from a problem in the production of the bile by the liver or an obstruction to its outflow via the gallbladder into the duodenum Pancreatic cancer may cause jaundice by growing to obstruct the outflow of the bile via the bile duct Jaundice always merits referral for investigation of its cause	**

A8: RED FLAGS OF DISEASES OF THE LIVER

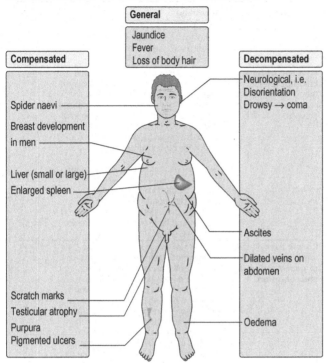

General
Jaundice
Fever
Loss of body hair

Compensated

Spider naevi

Breast development
in men

Liver (small or large)
Enlarged spleen

Scratch marks
Testicular atrophy
Purpura
Pigmented ulcers

Decompensated

Neurological, i.e.
Disorientation
Drowsy → coma

Ascites

Dilated veins on
abdomen

Oedema

Figure 2.3 The physical signs seen in cirrhosis of the liver (see A8.4). (From CTG Figure 3.1d-II.)

TABLE A8 Red flags of diseases of the liver

Red flag	Description	Reasoning	Priority
A8.1	**Jaundice:** yellowish skin, yellow whites of the eyes, and possibly dark urine and pale stools; itch may be a prominent symptom	Jaundice results from a problem in the production of the bile by the liver or an obstruction to its outflow via the gallbladder into the duodenum Jaundice may result from inflammation of the liver (hepatitis) or from liver cancer Hepatitis can be a result of infection (e.g. hepatitis A, B or C or glandular fever) and can also result from the inflammation caused by certain prescription medications and alcohol Jaundice always merits referral for investigation of its cause Viral hepatitis of any form is a notifiable disease[1]	**

TABLE A8 Continued

Red flag	Description	Reasoning	Priority
A8.2	**Right hypochondriac pain** (pain under the right ribs) with malaise for >3 days	This suggests liver or gallbladder pathology and should be considered for investigation, even in the absence of jaundice, if persisting for >3 days	**
A8.3	**Vomiting of fresh blood or altered blood** (looks like dark gravel or coffee grounds)	The appearance of blood in the vomit is always of concern as it is not possible to gauge the severity of bleeding and whether or not the bleeding is continuing. Refer if more than about a tablespoon of blood appears in the vomit (small amounts may simply be the result of a tear of the oesophagus lining during vomiting). There can be profuse bleeding from the base of the oesophagus in chronic liver disease, as distended varicose veins (varices) can rupture in this site. The patient in this situation can easily go into shock (see **A19.3**) and should be treated as an emergency	***
A8.4	**Known liver disease with the syndrome of oedema, bruising and confusion**	Liver disease may remain in a stable state for months to years, but the patient may become suddenly much more unwell once the disease has progressed to a certain point. This is the point at which the liver is no longer able to perform its function of the manufacture of blood proteins (including those necessary for blood clotting) and detoxification. Bruising, oedema and confusion can result (see Figure 2.3). This syndrome requires urgent medical management	**

[1]Notifiable diseases: notification of a number of specified infectious diseases is required of doctors in the UK as a statutory duty under the Public Health (Infectious Diseases) 1988 Act and the Public Health (Control of Diseases) 1988 Act and, more recently, the Health Protection (Notification) Regulations 2010. The UK Health Protection Agency (HPA) Centre for Infections collates details of each case of each disease that has been notified. This allows analyses of local and national trends. This is one example of a situation in which there is a legal requirement for a doctor to breach patient confidentiality.

Diseases that are notifiable include: acute encephalitis, acute poliomyelitis, acute infectious hepatitis, anthrax, cholera, diphtheria, enteric fevers (typhoid and paratyphoid), food poisoning, infectious bloody diarrhoea, leprosy, malaria, measles, meningitis (bacterial and viral forms), meningococcal septicaemia (without meningitis), mumps, plague, rabies, rubella, SARS, scarlet fever, smallpox, tetanus, tuberculosis, typhus, viral haemorrhagic fever, whooping cough and yellow fever.

A9: RED FLAGS OF DISEASES OF THE GALLBLADDER

TABLE A9 Red flags of diseases of the gallbladder

Red flag	Description	Reasoning	Priority
A9.1	**Jaundice:** yellowish skin, yellow whites of the eyes, and possibly dark urine and pale stools; itch may be a prominent symptom	Jaundice results from a problem in the production of the bile by the liver or an obstruction to its outflow via the gallbladder into the duodenum. Jaundice may result from sudden obstruction of the flow of bile by a gallstone. In this case it is usually accompanied by severe colicky pain (see **A6.8**). Jaundice can also develop slowly as a result of gradual obstruction by a tumour of the outflow of the gallbladder. Jaundice always merits referral for investigation of its cause	**
A9.2	**Right hypochondriac pain** (pain under the right ribs) with malaise for >3 days	This suggests liver or gallbladder pathology and should be considered for investigation, even in the absence of jaundice, if persisting for >3 days	**
A9.3	**Right hypochondriac pain** which is very intense and comes in waves. May be associated with fever and vomiting. May be associated with jaundice. This is one of the manifestations of the acute abdomen (see **A6.8**)	Obstruction of bile ducts by gallstones causes waves of intense pain as the duct attempts to contract against the obstruction. Fever and malaise can develop as the obstructed gallbladder becomes inflamed	**

A10: RED FLAGS OF DISEASES OF THE SMALL AND LARGE INTESTINES

TABLE A10 Red flags of diseases of the small and large intestines

Red flag	Description	Reasoning	Priority
A10.1	**Malabsorption syndrome:** loose pale stools and malnutrition; weight loss, thin hair, dry skin, cracked lips and peeled tongue Will present as failure to thrive in children	Malabsorption syndrome develops when there is an inability to absorb the nutrients in the diet, and weight loss and mineral and vitamin deficiencies result. Loose stools are the result of the presence of unabsorbed fat Disease of the small intestine (most commonly coeliac disease and Crohn's disease) can result in malabsorption syndrome Chronic pancreatitis is one of the causes of the malabsorption syndrome (see **A7.2**)	**/*
A10.2	**Diarrhoea with mucus or gripy pain** if not responding to treatment within a week	Persistent diarrhoea with mucus suggests either a serious episode of bowel infection or an episode of inflammatory bowel disease (Crohn's disease or ulcerative colitis) Both causes merit prompt referral for treatment Food poisoning and dysentery (severe bloody diarrhoea) are notifiable diseases (see **A6.2**)[1]	**
A10.3	**Onset of severe abdominal pain with collapse (the acute abdomen):** the pain can be constant or colicky (coming in waves); rigidity, guarding and rebound tenderness are serious signs	The 'acute abdomen' is a term that refers to the combination of severe abdominal pain together with an inability to continue with day-to-day activities ('collapse'). This syndrome can have benign causes, such as irritable bowel syndrome, dysmenorrhoea and ovulation pain, but needs high priority or urgent referral to exclude more serious conditions including appendicitis, perforated ulcer, peritonitis, obstructed bowel, pelvic inflammatory disease and gallstones Colicky pain indicates obstruction of a viscus (hollow organ) Rigidity of the abdomen, guarding (a reflex protective spasm of the abdominal muscles) and rebound tenderness (pain felt elsewhere in the abdomen when the pressure of the palpating hand is released) all suggest inflammation or perforation of a viscus Features of abdominal pain in children that suggest a more benign (functional) cause include mild pain that is worse in the morning, location of pain around the umbilicus and pain that is worse with anxiety	***/**

TABLE A10 Continued

Red flag	Description	Reasoning	Priority
A10.4	**Any episode of blood mixed in with stools**	Red blood mixed in with stools suggests bleeding from the lower part of the small intestine, the large intestine or rectum Possible causes are bowel infections, diverticulitis, inflammatory bowel disease (Crohn's disease or ulcerative colitis) and bowel cancer. All merit referral for investigation and treatment Acute infectious diarrhoea is a notifiable disease (see **A6.2**)[1] Blood that drips from the anus after defecation is common and is usually the result of haemorrhoids (piles). If the blood is not mixed in with the stools, the cause is likely to be benign	**
A10.5	**Signs of an inguinal hernia: swelling in the groin** that is more pronounced on standing, especially if uncomfortable	An inguinal hernia is the result of a weakness in the abdominal wall in the region of the inguinal crease (the groin). The abdominal contents can bulge into a narrow-necked passageway formed by this weakness, and this can be very uncomfortable An inguinal hernia carries the risk of a loop of bowel becoming obstructed, and then there is a risk of strangulation of that portion of the bowel. The patient should be referred for a surgical assessment of the risk of complications Refer as a high priority only if a hernia has become acutely very painful over the course of a few hours	*/**
A10.6	**Altered bowel habit** lasting for 3 weeks in someone >50 years old	Most people have a predictable pattern of defecation. If this pattern is broken for >3 weeks it may be a warning sign of inflammatory bowel disease or cancer. Consider referral in all people who develop this symptom over the age of 50 years because of the high risk of bowel cancer in this age group An increased frequency of defecation or increased mucus production are of particular concern	**/*

TABLE A10 Continued

Red flag	Description	Reasoning	Priority
A10.7	**Infectious bloody diarrhoea or food poisoning:** any episode of diarrhoea and vomiting in which food is suspected as the origin, or in which blood appears in the stools	Bloody diarrhoea which results from bacterial infection may manifest in profuse watery diarrhoea, abdominal cramps and blood in the stools. Clusters of related cases or a history of recent travel can suggest an infectious cause Food poisoning is the consequence of eating food which is contaminated with infectious organisms; it is commonly a result of poor food hygiene, together with insufficient cooking Both infectious bloody diarrhoea and food poisoning are notifiable diseases,[1] and as such merit referral so that they can be reported by a medical practitioner	**
A10.8	**Anal discharge/soiling with stool** (in underwear or bed)	Always refer for diagnosis if persistent and appearing in a previously continent child (could signify constipation with faecal overflow, a developmental problem of the bowel or emotional disturbance) An anal discharge may result from rectal or anal cancer, and in an elderly person a faecal discharge may result from constipation with overflow of faecal fluid. Both situations require referral	*/**
A10.9	**Painless lump felt in the anus**	This could be a benign skin tag or anal warts, and possibly may be an anal carcinoma. An undiagnosed anal lump needs referral for diagnosis if persisting for >2 weeks	*
A10.10	**Painful lump felt in the anus**	A painful anal lump could be a prolapsed haemorrhoid, a perianal haematoma (benign) or an anal carcinoma. It needs referral for diagnosis, and as high priority if pain is severe	**/*

TABLE A10 Continued

Red flag	Description	Reasoning	Priority
A10.11	Anal itch	A short history of intense nocturnal anal itch might be the result of threadworm infection A more prolonged history is most likely to be the result of haemorrhoids and skin tags. However, itch may result from the more serious conditions of lichen sclerosus or anal carcinoma, so should be referred for examination if not responding to simple treatment within 3 weeks	*

[1]Notifiable diseases: notification of a number of specified infectious diseases is required of doctors in the UK as a statutory duty under the Public Health (Infectious Diseases) 1988 Act and the Public Health (Control of Diseases) 1988 Act and, more recently, the Health Protection (Notification) Regulations 2010. The UK Health Protection Agency (HPA) Centre for Infections collates details of each case of each disease that has been notified. This allows analyses of local and national trends. This is one example of a situation in which there is a legal requirement for a doctor to breach patient confidentiality.

Diseases that are notifiable include: acute encephalitis, acute poliomyelitis, acute infectious hepatitis, anthrax, cholera, diphtheria, enteric fevers (typhoid and paratyphoid), food poisoning, infectious bloody diarrhoea, leprosy, malaria, measles, meningitis (bacterial and viral forms), meningococcal septicaemia (without meningitis), mumps, plague, rabies, rubella, SARS, scarlet fever, smallpox, tetanus, tuberculosis, typhus, viral haemorrhagic fever, whooping cough and yellow fever.

A11: RED FLAGS OF DISEASES OF THE BLOOD VESSELS

TABLE A11 Red flags of diseases of the blood vessels

Red flag	Description	Reasoning	Priority
A11.1	**Features of limb infarction:** suddenly extremely pale, painful, mottled and cold limb; if infarction is severe the limb may feel more numb than painful	Infarction results from the sudden obstruction of arterial blood supply to a limb, usually by a blood clot. The patient requires urgent referral for surgical removal of the obstruction	***

TABLE A11 Continued

Red flag	Description	Reasoning	Priority
A11.2	**Features of severely compromised circulation to the extremities:** • pain in the calf that is related to exercise and relieved by rest • pain in the calf in bed at night, relieved by hanging the leg out of bed (i.e. not cramp) • cold, purplish shiny skin • areas of blackened skin (gangrene)	If obstruction to the arterial circulation is gradual and/or partial, the pain will only appear when oxygen demands are higher than normal. Pain may appear on exercise and in bed, and there will be changes on the skin of the affected limb that suggest chronic (long-standing) poor circulation. There is a high risk of infarction and also of progressive gangrene, which could lead to the need for amputation. These symptoms require referral for assessment, lifestyle advice (especially advice on smoking cessation) and consideration for vascular surgery	**/*
A11.3	**Features of an aortic aneurysm:** pulsatile mass in abdomen >5 cm in diameter. (Usually affects people >50 years old and is associated with the degenerative changes of atherosclerosis)	The aorta is palpable in the abdomen as a pulsatile tube of about 2 cm in diameter. In the case of aneurysm, the width of this tube increases, and a palpable width of >5 cm merits assessment by ultrasonography so that the risk of rupture can be formally assessed Early treatment of high-risk cases is life-saving Refer urgently if abdominal or central back pain develops with a coexistent aortic aneurysm (see **A11.4**)	* and *** if pain develops
A11.4	**Features of a ruptured aortic aneurysm:** acute abdominal or back pain, with collapse; features of shock may be coexistent. This is one of the manifestations of the acute abdomen (see **A6.8**)	A rupture of an aortic aneurysm is an emergency situation and the patient needs urgent surgical treatment A rupture may be presaged by abdominal discomfort or back pain, so if these develop in the presence of a suspected aneurysm refer as a matter of high priority/urgency	***
A11.5	**Features of meningococcal septicaemia:** acute onset of a purpuric rash, possibly accompanied by headache, vomiting and fever	The purpuric rash in meningococcal septicaemia is a result of vasculitis (inflammation of the blood vessels). This is a serious warning sign of a devastating disease process, and the patient requires urgent referral for antibiotic treatment Meningococcal septicaemia is a notifiable disease[1]	***

TABLE A11 Continued

Red flag	Description	Reasoning	Priority
A11.6	**Features of severe consequences of varicose veins:** broken or itchy skin close to the veins indicates a risk of varicose ulcer	Varicose veins are usually benign, but can reduce the effectiveness of the drainage of blood from the affected area. This can result in weakened, dry and itchy (eczematous) skin. A break to the skin can easily develop into an ulcer (See Figure 2.4) and in this situation would merit referral for assessment and nursing care Thrombophlebitis (inflammation of a length of a varicose vein) need not be referred if localised and superficial	*
A11.7	**Features of a deep venous thrombosis (DVT):** a hot swollen tender calf, can be accompanied by fever and malaise. There is an increased risk after air travel and surgery, and in pregnancy, cancer and if on oral contraceptive pill	DVT develops slowly and needs to be distinguished from gastrocnemius muscle strain (redness would be minimal and no fever) and thrombophlebitis (redness localised to the path of a varicose vein) If DVT is suspected it merits high-priority referral, as without anticoagulant treatment there is a risk of pulmonary embolism (blood clot breaking off to lodge in the arterial circulation of the lungs). The patient should be advised to refrain from unnecessary exercise until he or she has been medically assessed	**

[1]Notifiable diseases: notification of a number of specified infectious diseases is required of doctors in the UK as a statutory duty under the Public Health (Infectious Diseases) 1988 Act and the Public Health (Control of Diseases) 1988 Act and, more recently, the Health Protection (Notification) Regulations 2010. The UK Health Protection Agency (HPA) Centre for Infections collates details of each case of each disease that has been notified. This allows analyses of local and national trends. This is one example of a situation in which there is a legal requirement for a doctor to breach patient confidentiality.

Diseases that are notifiable include: acute encephalitis, acute poliomyelitis, acute infectious hepatitis, anthrax, cholera, diphtheria, enteric fevers (typhoid and paratyphoid), food poisoning, infectious bloody diarrhoea, leprosy, malaria, measles, meningitis (bacterial and viral forms), meningococcal septicaemia (without meningitis), mumps, plague, rabies, rubella, SARS, scarlet fever, smallpox, tetanus, tuberculosis, typhus, viral haemorrhagic fever, whooping cough and yellow fever.

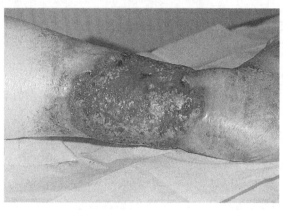

Figure 2.4 Varicose ulcer of the inner aspect of the lower leg (see A11.6). (From CTG Figure 3.2c-III.)

A12: RED FLAGS OF HYPERTENSION

TABLE A12 Red flags of hypertension

Red flag	Description	Reasoning	Priority
A12.1	**Features of malignant hypertension:** diastolic pressure >120 mmHg with symptoms, including recently worsening headaches, blurred vision, chest pain	At a certain level, hypertension leads to a negative cycle of increasing vascular damage and worsening hypertension. This is malignant hypertension, which carries a high risk of stroke and other cardiovascular events. Visual disturbances and headaches are serious signs	***/**
A12.2	**Seriously high hypertension:** • systolic pressure ≥220 mmHg • diastolic pressure ≥120 mmHg • no symptoms	Refer as a high priority. Current medical guidelines[1] state that immediate medical management is required to prevent stroke or other cardiovascular events	**

TABLE A12 Continued

Red flag	Description	Reasoning	Priority
A12.3	**Severe hypertension:** • systolic pressure ≥180 mmHg • diastolic pressure ≥110 mmHg	Refer if not responding to your treatment in 2 weeks, or straight away if major risk factors are present[2] Current medical guidelines[1] recommend medical treatment if there is no improvement in the blood pressure within 2 weeks	*
A12.4	**Moderate hypertension:** • systolic pressure ≥160 mmHg and <180 mmHg • diastolic pressure ≥100 mmHg and <110 mmHg	Refer if not responding to your treatment within 4 weeks, or straight away for medical assessment if major risk factors are present[2] Current medical guidelines[1] recommend medical management if there is no improvement over 4–12 weeks, and within 4 weeks if risk factors are present In those over 80 years old, the threshold for treatment, if no risk factors are present, is less stringent: treatment is advised if blood pressure exceeds 160/90 mmHg, and has been sustained for 3–6 months	*
A12.5	**Mild hypertension:** • systolic pressure ≥140 mmHg and <160 mmHg • diastolic pressure ≥90 mmHg and <100 mmHg	Refer for treatment if major risk factors[2] are present and if there is no improvement within 3 months If no major risk factors are present, refer only if you suspect that the cardiovascular risk is increased because of the presence of other risk factors, such as smoking or hyperlipidaemia In people >80 years old, the threshold for treatment if no risk factors are present is less stringent: treatment is advised if blood pressure exceeds 160/90 mmHg, and has been sustained for 3–6 months	*
A12.6	**Hypertension of any level with diabetes**	Always refer for medical management, as the conventional medical opinion is that blood pressure should be maintained below 130/80 mmHg in people with diabetes because of the much greater risk of vascular and renal complications	**/*
A12.7	**Hypertension of any level with established kidney disease**	Always refer for medical management, as blood pressure should be maintained below 130/80 mmHg in people with kidney disease because of the much greater risk of worsening kidney damage	**/*

TABLE A12 Continued

Red flag	Description	Reasoning	Priority
A12.8	**Hypertension of any level in pregnancy** (see A37.9–A37.11)	Always refer because of the increased risk of pre-eclampsia and placental damage	**

[1]Advice in this table is based on the chapter on cardiovascular diseases in the September 2011 version of the *British National Formulary* (RSPG), which takes into account the recommendations of the Joint British Societies (JBS2: British Societies' guidelines on prevention of cardiovascular disease in clinical practice, *Heart* 2005;91(Suppl V):v1–v52). Tables for calculating cardiovascular risk on the basis of risk factors can be found in this supplement.

[2]In this case, *major risk factors* are features that are known to be associated with increased risk of a cardiovascular event in the presence of hypertension. These include *diabetes, past history of heart disease, chronic leg ischaemia* and *kidney disease*.

Medical doctors now use risk factor calculation tables to predict more accurately the statistical risk in an individual case and this can help with decision making about whether or not medication is appropriate. *Other risk factors*, such as sex, age, smoking status and lipid levels, will be taken into account in such calculations. Medication is considered advisable in those for whom the 10-year risk of a cardiovascular event is predicted to be more than 20%. For this reason, referral is advised for risk assessment if any of the risk factors mentioned above are present or suspected to be present. Therefore, for example, if lipid levels are not known, referral should be considered. Risk calculation can help a patient make a more informed decision about the potential benefits of medication, and may also help them make the decision to adjust their lifestyle to improve their risk status. In line with current medical wisdom, all patients with hypertension may benefit from advice on lifestyle changes to reduce blood pressure or cardiovascular risk. Relevant lifestyle changes include smoking cessation, weight reduction, reduction of excessive alcohol intake, reduction of dietary salt, reduction of total and saturated fat in diet, increasing exercise and increasing fruit and vegetable intake.

A13: RED FLAGS OF ANGINA AND HEART ATTACK

TABLE A13 Red flags of angina and heart attack

Red flag	Description	Reasoning	Priority
A13.1	**Features of stable angina:** central chest pain related to exertion, eating or the cold and which improves with rest. Pain is heavy, gripping (rather than sharp or stabbing). It can radiate down the neck and arms *Beware*: can present as episodes of breathlessness/chest tightness but without pain in the elderly	Chest pain is a common anxiety symptom, and also is a common feature of peptic ulcer disease, hiatus hernia and oesophagitis. Stable angina is distinguished from these syndromes by being predictably related to exertion, and generally develops in those over 35 years old. It is far more likely to develop in older people and those with cardiovascular risk factors (see footnotes to **A12**). If there is any doubt it is advisable to refer for assessment, as angina carries a high risk of heart attack and other cardiovascular events	**/*

TABLE A13 Continued

Red flag	Description	Reasoning	Priority
A13.2	**Features of unstable angina or heart attack:** sustained intense chest pain associated with fear or dread. Palpitations and breathlessness may be present. The patient may vomit or develop a cold sweat *Beware*: can present as sudden onset of breathlessness, palpitations or confusion but without pain in the elderly	Very intense and heavy chest pain that tends to radiate to the left shoulder and arm is suggestive of cardiac pain. If sustained, this is a situation in which there is a high risk of cardiac arrest or worsening cardiovascular damage. Keep the patient calm, upright and still while waiting for help to arrive Under UK Health and Safety Executive guidance,[1] qualified first aiders are permitted to administer aspirin in the situation of suspected heart attack. There is very strong clinical evidence to support the benefits of aspirin in reducing the risk of fatal complications, and this effect is more powerful the sooner the aspirin is given. The patient should be offered one 300 mg tablet to be chewed or swallowed. Aspirin is contraindicated in children <12 years old, in pregnancy, if the patient has a bleeding disorder or is on anticoagulant medication, and in cases where there is a known allergy to aspirin or aspirin-induced asthma NB: Chest pain is a common anxiety symptom and also is a common feature of peptic ulcer disease, hiatus hernia and oesophagitis. If associated with anxiety it is more likely to be centrally located and be sharp in quality	Consider aspirin treatment as soon as possible ***
A13.3	**Sudden-onset tearing chest pain with radiation to the back:** features of shock may be present (faintness, low blood pressure, rapid pulse)	This intense, acute form of chest pain is suggestive of a dissecting aortic aneurysm. In this case, urgent referral is required, but aspirin should not be given as it promotes bleeding	***

[1]For the UK Health and Safety Executive guidance on first aid at work and the administration of aspirin, go to http://www.hse.gov.uk/firstaid/faqs.htm.

A14: RED FLAGS OF HEART FAILURE AND ARRHYTHMIAS

TABLE A14 Red flags of heart failure and arrhythmias

Red flag	Description	Reasoning	Priority
A14.1	**Features of mild, chronic heart failure:** slight swelling of the ankles, slight breathlessness on exertion and when lying flat, cough and with no palpitations or chest pain Dry cough may be the only symptom in sedentary elderly people	In chronic heart failure, the pumping ability of the heart is reduced, and this results in accumulation of tissue fluid in the lungs (breathlessness) and ankles (oedema). It may remain undiagnosed if mild, but it is associated with increased risk of worsening damage to the heart Current medical guidance is that all patients will benefit in terms of reduced symptoms and increased life-expectancy from medical treatment of heart failure, and referral is recommended for assessment by electrocardiography and echocardiography	*
A14.2	**Features of severe chronic heart failure:** marked swelling of the ankles and lower legs, disabling breathlessness and exhaustion	Severe chronic heart failure is a serious condition associated with a high mortality. It will benefit from medical management, and this is associated with an improved life-expectancy	**
A14.3	**Features of acute heart failure:** sudden onset of disabling breathlessness, and watery cough	Acute heart failure results from a sudden loss in the ability of the heart to pump effectively, and most commonly results from heart attack, arrhythmia or valve damage. The patient requires emergency treatment and needs to be kept calm and sitting upright until help arrives	***
A14.4	**An irregularly irregular pulse** (possible atrial fibrillation)	An irregularly irregular (totally unpredictable) pulse is a feature of atrial fibrillation. This arrhythmia carries a risk of the production of tiny blood clots within the chaotically contracting atria of the heart. These clots may then be dispersed (as emboli) to lodge in the circulation of the brain, and so carry a risk of transient ischaemic attack and stroke Refer in all cases for further assessment, and as a high priority if features of heart failure or angina are also present, or if there is a history of blackouts or neurological symptoms	**/*

TABLE A14 Continued

Red flag	Description	Reasoning	Priority
A14.5	**A very rapid pulse of 140–250 beats/ minute** (most likely to be supraventricular tachycardia or atrial fibrillation)	Episodes of tachycardia (very rapid pulse) can be exhausting for the patient, and may progress to a more serious arrhythmia or lead to the symptoms of acute heart failure If the attack is not settling in 5 minutes, refer urgently for medical management. If the attack settles, refer as a high priority so that the cause can be investigated	***/**
A14.6	**A very slow pulse of 40–50 beats/minute** (complete heart block), either of recent onset or associated with features such as dizziness, light-headedness or fainting	Some healthy individuals have a naturally slow heart rate, particularly if they have trained as athletes. However, if the rate suddenly drops to 40–50 beats/minute, this is characteristic of an arrhythmia called 'complete heart block', in which the natural pacemaker of the heart becomes unable to transmit a more frequent impulse to the ventricles. In this case, the patient will start to feel dizzy and breathless, and may pass out. Refer urgently if ongoing, and as a high priority if the attack has settled down. The patient will need assessment for the implant of a pacemaker system	***/**
A14.7	**A pulse that is regular but skips beats at regular intervals** (i.e. 1 out of every 3–5 beats is missing) (incomplete heart block)	The occasional missed beat (ventricular ectopic) is not a worrying finding. It is more likely to occur in older people However, if the beat is missed at a regular and frequent rate (more often than 1 in every 5 beats), this suggests a conduction defect called 'incomplete heart block', which carries a risk of progression to a more serious arrhythmia, and merits referral for cardiological assessment If the patient is well and was unaware of the problem until you found it, refer non-urgently	*
A14.8	**Unexplained falls or faints** in an elderly person	These may be the result of an arrhythmia (cardiac syncope). A temporary cardiac arrhythmia may result in a dizzy spell or sudden loss of consciousness from which an elderly person may recover very quickly. These episodes may account for unexplained falls. Consider referral if a patient reports a fall but cannot remember how it happened	**/*

TABLE A14 Continued

Red flag	Description	Reasoning	Priority
A14.9	**Cardiac arrest:** collapse with no palpable pulse	Cardiac arrest results from the arrhythmia known as 'ventricular fibrillation (VF)'. The most common cause is heart attack (myocardial infarction), but VF can also occur spontaneously as a result of degenerative damage to the conducting system of the heart. VF may also result from electric shock	***
		In contrast to atrial fibrillation, in which the heart continues to pump fairly efficiently, when the ventricles of the heart go into chaotic rhythm the pumping function of the heart is totally lost and there is immediate circulatory collapse. Once help has been called, the patient requires urgent cardiopulmonary resuscitation from a qualified first aider	

A15: RED FLAGS OF PERICARDITIS

TABLE A15 Red flags of pericarditis

Red flag	Description	Reasoning	Priority
A15.1	**Features of uncomplicated pericarditis:** sharp central chest pain that is worse on leaning forward and lying down. Fever should be slight and the pulse rate ≤100 beats/minute. Complications include: • features of heart failure (breathlessness and oedema) • features of arrhythmia (tachycardia) • symptoms of heart attack/unstable angina	Pericarditis can result from a viral infection or as part of a complex metabolic illness such as renal failure. It can also complicate recovery from a heart attack In its uncomplicated form the patient will have central chest pain that is affected by posture and other chest movements. If pericarditis is suspected, it is advisable to refer for further cardiac investigations in hospital, as the condition can deteriorate and affect the rhythm or pumping capacity of the heart Refer urgently if complications are apparent	**

A16: RED FLAGS OF UPPER RESPIRATORY DISEASE

TABLE A16 Red flags of upper respiratory disease

Red flag	Description	Reasoning	Priority
A16.1	**Features of progressive upper respiratory infection in susceptible people** (e.g. the frail elderly, the immunocompromised and people with pre-existing lower respiratory disease): cough and fever or new production of yellow–green phlegm, each persisting for >3 days	In healthy people, an upper respiratory infection (i.e. affecting any part of the respiratory tract above and including the bronchi) may be protracted but is not necessarily a serious condition. In most cases, as long as there is no breathlessness or the patient is not a smoker, it is safe to treat conservatively and there is no need for antibiotics In healthy people, consider referral if there is no response to your treatment within 1–2 weeks However, in the elderly and the immunocompromised (including those with chronic diseases such as cancer, kidney failure and AIDS), severe infections can be masked by relatively minor symptoms, and it is advisable to refer any respiratory condition that persists for >3 days People with pre-existing lung disease (e.g. asthma, chronic bronchitis, emphysema, lung cancer, cystic fibrosis) are at increased risk of progressive infection, and similarly merit early referral Smokers commonly do not recover as quickly from upper respiratory infections and early antibiotic treatment may be merited in this case also	**
A16.2	**Features of progression of infection to the lower respiratory tract:** moderate to severe breathlessness[1] with malaise suggests the involvement of the bronchi or lower air passages. Usually accompanied by cough and fever, but may be the only symptom of an infection in the elderly or immunocompromised	Even in healthy people, an infection that descends to below the bronchi is a more serious condition, as the ability of the lungs to exchange carbon dioxide and oxygen will be compromised by the narrowing of the thin airways of the bronchioles and inflammation of the alveoli (air sacs) Breathlessness is a feature of lower respiratory tract narrowing or infection and should be taken seriously, especially in the elderly immunocompromised and those with pre-existing lung disease (e.g. asthma, chronic bronchitis, emphysema, lung cancer, cystic fibrosis) and smokers All patients with breathlessness resulting from lung infection should be referred for a high priority assessment by a medical doctor A respiratory rate of >30 breaths/minute is a marker of significant breathlessness	***/**

TABLE A16 Continued

Red flag	Description	Reasoning	Priority
A16.3	**A single, grossly enlarged tonsil:** if the patient is unwell and feverish and has foul-smelling breath, this suggests quinsy	Quinsy is the development of an abscess in the tonsil. It carries a serious risk of obstruction of the airways and requires a same-day surgical opinion Refer urgently if the patient is experiencing any restriction of breathing (stridor may be heard: see **A16.5**)	***/**
A16.4	**A single, grossly enlarged tonsil:** if the patient appears well, lymphoma is a possible diagnosis	If the patient appears well, you need to consider that a single enlarged tonsil in a young person may, very rarely, result from a lymphoma and should be referred for exclusion of this diagnosis. However, grossly enlarged tonsils are not an uncommon finding in someone who has suffered from recurrent tonsillitis. In this case the tonsils are usually bilaterally enlarged	*
A16.5	**Stridor** (harsh, noisy breathing heard on both the inbreath and the outbreath)	Stridor is a noise that suggests upper airways obstruction. It is a serious red flag if it develops suddenly. It suggests possible swelling of the air passages due to laryngotracheitis, quinsy or epiglottitis If restriction to breathing is significant, the patient with stridor will be sitting very still It is important not to ask to see the tongue, as this can affect the position of the epiglottis, and may worsen the obstruction Exposing the patient to steam (from a nearby kettle or running shower) can alleviate swelling while waiting for help to arrive	***/**
A16.6	**Any new onset of difficulty in breathing in a small child** (<8 years old), including unexplained blockage of nostril	Always take a new onset of difficulty in breathing in a child seriously, and refer for medical assessment to exclude serious disease. Possible common causes include lower respiratory infections, asthma, allergic reactions, inhalation of foreign bodies and congenital heart disease	***/**
A16.7	**An unexplained persistent blockage of the nostril** on one side in an adult (for >3 weeks)	One-sided blockage of a nostril is unusual in benign conditions (e.g. nasal polyposis). It may be the presenting sign of a carcinoma of the nasopharynx. A one-sided bloody discharge is a warning sign of this	**/*

[1]Categorisation of respiratory rate in adults:

– Normal respiratory rate in an adult: 10–20 breaths/minute (one breath is one inhalation and exhalation).
– Moderate breathlessness in an adult: >30 breaths/minute.
– Severe breathlessness in an adult: >60 breaths/minute.

TABLE A16 Continued

Categorisation of respiratory rate in children:

– The normal range for respiratory rate in children varies according to age.
– The following rates indicate moderate to severe breathlessness:

newborn (0–3 months)	>60 breaths/minute
infant (3 months to 2 years)	>50 breaths/minute
young child (2–8 years)	>40 breaths/minute
older child to adult	>30 breaths/minute

A17: RED FLAGS OF LOWER RESPIRATORY DISEASE

TABLE A17 Red flags of lower respiratory disease

Red flag	Description	Reasoning	Priority
A17.1	**Features of progressive upper respiratory infection in susceptible people** (e.g. the frail elderly, the immunocompromised and people with pre-existing disease of the bronchi and bronchioles): cough and fever or new production of yellow–green phlegm, each persisting for >3 days	In healthy people, an upper respiratory infection (i.e. affecting any part of the respiratory tract above and including the bronchi) may be protracted, but is not necessarily a serious condition. In most cases, as long as there is no breathlessness, it is safe to treat conservatively, and there is no need for antibiotics In healthy people, consider referral if there is no response to your treatment within 1–2 weeks However, in the elderly and the immunocompromised (including those with chronic diseases such as cancer, kidney failure and AIDS), severe infections can be masked by relatively minor symptoms, and it is advisable to refer any respiratory condition that persists for >3 days People with pre-existing lung disease (e.g. asthma, chronic bronchitis, emphysema, lung cancer, cystic fibrosis) are at increased risk of progressive infection, and similarly merit early referral Smokers commonly do not recover as quickly from upper respiratory infections and early antibiotic treatment may be merited in this case also	**

TABLE A17 Continued

Red flag	Description	Reasoning	Priority
A17.2	**Any new onset of difficulty in breathing in a young child** (<8 years old)	Always take a new onset of difficulty in breathing in a child seriously, and refer for medical assessment to exclude serious disease. Common causes include lower respiratory infections, asthma, allergic reactions, inhalation of foreign bodies and congenital heart disease	***/**
A17.3	**Features of severe asthma:** at least two of the following: • rapidly worsening breathlessness • >30 respirations/minute (or more if a child)[1] • heart rate >110 beats/minute • reluctance to talk because of breathlessness • need to sit upright and still to assist breathing • central cyanosis (see **A17.12**) is a very serious sign	Severe asthma is a potentially life-threatening condition and may develop in someone who has no previous history of severe attacks. Urgent referral is required so that medical management of the attack can be instigated. Keep the patient as calm as possible while waiting for help to arrive It may be very difficult to differentiate an asthma attack from the more benign situation of panic attack (characterised by a felt experience of intense fear, racing heart, increased depth of breathing, numbness and tingling of the extremities, and mild muscle spasms), and it is possible for the two to coincide, as an experience of breathlessness can trigger a panic reaction. In this situation, the key feature is respiratory rate, and if this does not respond to calming measures within a few minutes, and rebreathing exhaled carbon dioxide (by breathing into a paper bag) within a minute or two, referral needs to be considered. Central cyanosis would never be apparent in a panic attack, so if present this is an absolute indicator for urgent referral	***
A17.4	**Haemoptysis:** any episode of coughing up of more than a teaspoon of blood	Blood-streaked sputum is a common and benign occurrence in upper respiratory tract infections, and is not a reason for referral if the amount of blood is small and infection is self-limiting (i.e. episode limited to the few days when cough from the infection is present) A larger amount of fresh blood may herald more serious bleeding in those with bronchiectasis. Also, it may be the first symptom of lung cancer or tuberculosis. Blood in the sputum also occurs in the case of pulmonary embolism	**

TABLE A17 Continued

Red flag	Description	Reasoning	Priority
A17.5	**New onset of chronic cough or deep, persistent chest pain in a smoker**	The most common first symptom of lung cancer is a chronic, irritating cough, which may feel different to the clearing of phlegm that characterises the smoker's cough Rarely, lung cancer can cause deep, persistent chest pain, but this is a less usual first symptom	**/*
A17.6	**Unexplained hoarseness** lasting for >3 weeks: may be the first symptom of laryngeal or lung cancer (particularly in smokers >50 years old)	Prolonged hoarseness is usually benign in origin and may be diagnosed as chronic laryngitis. This painless syndrome is commonly the result of misuse or overuse of the vocal cords However, the possibility of laryngeal cancer in smokers >50 years old needs to be considered Lung cancer can also be a cause of hoarseness, as the recurrent laryngeal nerve that passes deep in the chest can be damaged by an infiltrating tumour. Again smokers >50 years old are a high-risk group Referral is advised to exclude these less likely possible causes of chronic hoarseness	*
A17.7	**Features of infection of the alveoli (pneumonia).** Features include: • cough • fever • malaise • >30 respirations/minute (or more if a child)[1] • heart rate >110 beats/minute • reluctance to talk because of breathlessness • need to sit upright and still to assist breathing • cyanosis (see **A17.12**) is a very serious sign	Pneumonia means that inflammation (usually as a result of infection) has descended to the level of the air sacs (alveoli) in the lungs. As these sacs are involved in the exchange of gases, breathlessness is always part of the picture of pneumonia. As the infection is so deep, the patient can become extremely unwell and may need hospital treatment Use the severity of the symptoms to guide the urgency of the referral Severe breathlessness merits urgent referral	***/**

TABLE A17 Continued

Red flag	Description	Reasoning	Priority
A17.8	**Features of pleurisy:** localised chest pain that is associated with inspiration and expiration. Refer if associated with fever and breathlessness, as this is an indication of associated pneumonia	Pleurisy is the syndrome resulting from inflammation of a region of the pleural lining of the lungs. Inflammation of the pleural lining leads to a localised region of chest-wall pain, which worsens with coughing and breathing in Pleurisy commonly results from a viral infection and in this case may be a benign syndrome associated with no other lung damage However, pleurisy may be a complication of the spread of pneumonia to the periphery of a lung, in which case it would be associated with malaise and breathlessness Pleurisy can also result from non-infectious causes, such as pulmonary embolism, in which case there will be breathlessness and sometimes expectoration of bloody sputum (see **A17.10**) If clearly associated with an upper respiratory infection and if there is no breathlessness, there is no need for immediate referral. However, a patient with pleurisy will need to be referred if the symptom is not settling within 1–2 days	If associated with breathlessness **
A17.9	**Features of tuberculosis infection:** chronic productive cough, weight loss, night sweats, blood in sputum for >2 weeks	Tuberculosis is more common in people who have lived in countries where tuberculosis is endemic, and in those who live in situations of poverty and in overcrowded damp conditions. It can also develop in people who have close contact with those at high risk Referral is for isolation, diagnosis and initiation of a prolonged programme of antibiotic therapy. Contacts will be traced and tested for infection if the diagnosis is confirmed Tuberculosis is a notifiable disease[2]	**

TABLE A17 Continued

Red flag	Description	Reasoning	Priority
A17.10	**Features of pulmonary embolism:** sudden onset of pleurisy (see **A17.8**) with breathlessness, cyanosis (see **A17.12**), collapse	Pulmonary embolism is the result of a lodging of a blood clot or multiple blood clots (emboli) in the arterial circulation supplying the lungs (pulmonary circulation). If the blood clot is large, there can be a sudden reduction in the oxygenation power of the lung, and this can result in collapse and sudden death. In less severe cases, the infarction of the lung tissue manifests as pleurisy with breathlessness, and blood may be coughed up in the sputum This syndrome merits urgent referral for anticoagulation (thinning of the blood)	***
A17.11	**Features of sudden lung collapse (pneumothorax):** onset of severe breathlessness; there may be some pleurisy (see **A17.8**) and collapse if very severe	Pneumothorax can occur spontaneously, or may be provoked by a puncture of the lungs. It is notorious among acupuncturists as a recognised complication of needling vulnerable points in the thorax, and practitioners should be vigilant that in extremely rare cases the symptoms can develop gradually up to 24 hours after a needle puncture	***
A17.12	**Central cyanosis** (as a new finding)	Cyanosis describes the blue colouring that appears when the blood is poorly oxygenated. The oxygen saturation of the blood needs to be less than 85% for cyanosis to become apparent. (The normal saturation level of the blood is >98%) Cyanosis of the extremities is a common finding in extreme cold and is not necessarily a serious sign. It is the result of sluggish circulation in the peripheral tissues, but does not necessarily indicate a generally depleted level of oxygen in the blood Central cyanosis from poor oxygenation can be seen on the tongue and in the complexion. Central cyanosis is a very serious sign that the body is failing to maintain adequate blood oxygen levels It can be the result of respiratory disease or cardiac disease, in which case there will be associated breathlessness. It also can result from respiratory suppression (for example with drugs or neurological disease), in which case the respiratory rate may be lower than normal Some people with chronic lung or heart disease may demonstrate central cyanosis yet be in a stable state However, if cyanosis is found in an acutely ill patient then this merits urgent referral	***

TABLE A17 Continued

[1]Categorisation of respiratory rate in adults:

– Normal respiratory rate in an adult: 10–20 breaths/minute (one breath is one inhalation and exhalation).
– Moderate breathlessness in an adult: >30 breaths/minute.
– Severe breathlessness in an adult: >60 breaths/minute.

Categorisation of respiratory rate in children:

– The normal range for respiratory rate in children varies according to age.
– The following rates indicate moderate to severe breathlessness:

newborn (0–3 months)	>60 breaths/minute
infant (3 months to 2 years)	>50 breaths/minute
young child (2–8 years)	>40 breaths/minute
older child to adult	>30 breaths/minute

[2]Notifiable diseases: notification of a number of specified infectious diseases is required of doctors in the UK as a statutory duty under the Public Health (Infectious Diseases) 1988 Act and the Public Health (Control of Diseases) 1988 Act and, more recently, the Health Protection (Notification) Regulations 2010. The UK Health Protection Agency (HPA) Centre for Infections collates details of each case of each disease that has been notified. This allows analyses of local and national trends. This is one example of a situation in which there is a legal requirement for a doctor to breach patient confidentiality.

Diseases that are notifiable include: acute encephalitis, acute poliomyelitis, acute infectious hepatitis, anthrax, cholera, diphtheria, enteric fevers (typhoid and paratyphoid), food poisoning, infectious bloody diarrhoea, leprosy, malaria, measles, meningitis (bacterial and viral forms), meningococcal septicaemia (without meningitis), mumps, plague, rabies, rubella, SARS, scarlet fever, smallpox, tetanus, tuberculosis, typhus, viral haemorrhagic fever, whooping cough and yellow fever.

A18: RED FLAGS OF ANAEMIA

TABLE A18 Red flags of anaemia

Red flag	Description	Reasoning	Priority
A18.1	**Features of long-standing anaemia:** any of the general symptoms of anaemia should be considered as a reason for referral so that serious treatable causes can be excluded. These include: • pallor • tiredness • palpitations • breathlessness on exertion • feeling of faintness • depression • sore mouth and tongue	'Anaemia' refers to a reduced haemoglobin level in the blood. Haemoglobin is the iron-containing pigment that enables red blood cells to carry high concentrations of oxygen to the tissues. When haemoglobin levels are low, the tissues experience relative oxygen lack Reduced concentration of the pigment in the blood can be seen in the skin as pallor The cardiovascular system responds by increasing the heart rate and the respiratory rate increases, so leading to palpitations and breathlessness Iron stores in the body become low as iron is utilised to the maximum, and the tissue cells suffer, meaning that the person suffers tiredness, depression and sore mouth and tongue, and dry skin and hair Referral is important to establish the cause of the anaemia Causes include: • increased blood loss (particularly from menstruation and bleeding from stomach or bowel, and prolonged use of aspirin or non-steroidal anti-inflammatory drugs) • reduced production of blood in the marrow (due to poor diet, malabsorption of iron, vitamin B_{12} or folic acid from the diet, and bone marrow disease) • chronic illness Mild anaemia is common and benign in pregnancy	**/*

TABLE A18 Continued

Red flag	Description	Reasoning	Priority
A18.2	**Features of severe anaemia:** the following additional symptoms and signs suggest that anaemia is very severe: • extreme tiredness • severe breathlessness on exertion • excessive bruising • severe visual disturbances • chest pain on exertion • tachycardia • oedema	(See **A18.1**.) Severe anaemia puts extra strain on the heart as it attempts to increase oxygen delivery to the tissues by increasing cardiac output. This can lead to cardiac failure and angina	**
A18.3	**Features of pernicious anaemia:** • tiredness • lemon-yellow pallor • gradual onset of neurological symptoms (numbness, weakness)	Pernicious anaemia is a form of anaemia that results from an impaired ability to absorb vitamin B_{12} from the digestive tract. The underlying cause is an auto-immune disease that affects the production of a protein (intrinsic factor) from the stomach. Intrinsic factor needs to bind to vitamin B_{12} before the vitamin can be absorbed As vitamin B_{12} is also vital to the health of the nervous system, neurological symptoms can develop if deficiency is prolonged. Treatment involves regular and lifelong injections of vitamin B_{12}	**/*

A19: RED FLAGS OF HAEMORRHAGE AND SHOCK

TABLE A19 Red flags of haemorrhage and shock

Red flag	Description	Reasoning	Priority
A19.1	**Continuing blood loss:** any situation in which significant bleeding is continuing for more than a few minutes without any signs of abating (except in the context of menstruation)	An adequate volume of blood in the circulation is essential to maintain the blood pressure required to enable adequate perfusion of the organs and tissues of the body. If the blood pressure drops too low, the syndrome of shock develops (see A19.3) Shock is defined as a situation in which there is a failure of the circulatory system to maintain adequate perfusion of vital organs If bleeding is continuing unabated the patient needs to be referred for fluid replacement and medical or surgical intervention to prevent further blood loss. This is of particular concern if the bleeding is from an internal location Administer basic first aid to accessible bleeding sites while waiting for help to arrive	★★★
A19.2	**Features of severe blood loss leading to shock:** refer if blood has been lost and the following symptoms and signs have been present for more than a few minutes or are worsening: • dizziness, fainting and confusion • rapid pulse of >100 beats/minute • blood pressure <90/50 mmHg • cold and clammy extremities	If the symptoms of shock (see A19.3) are developing this is an emergency situation. Administer basic first aid to bleeding sites. Ensure the patient is lying down and is kept warm while waiting for help to arrive	★★★

TABLE A19 Continued

Red flag	Description	Reasoning	Priority
A19.3	**General symptoms of shock:** • dizziness, fainting and confusion • rapid pulse of >100 beats/minute • blood pressure <90/50 mmHg • cold and clammy extremities Refer if these symptoms are worsening or sustained (more than a few seconds)	Shock can result from: • blood loss and extreme dehydration (hypovolaemic shock) • an allergic reaction (anaphylactic shock) • overwhelming infection (endotoxic shock) • failure of the heart to maintain an adequate circulation (cardiogenic shock resulting from damage to heart muscle, heart valves or from an arrhythmia) Sustained shock is always a situation in which treatment is required as an emergency, as the vulnerable organs of the brain, kidneys and heart are at risk of damage from inadequate levels of oxygen and nutrients A faint can produce a syndrome that is akin to shock, but the drop in blood pressure is always short lived and the person should start to recover within seconds. In the case of a faint, the drop in blood pressure follows a sudden slowing of the heart rate. For this reason, a weak and slow pulse would be expected in the few seconds following a faint, and this should return to a normal rate within 1–2 minutes. There is no need to refer in this situation	*** Unless faint is a likely diagnosis (i.e. patient starts recovering within seconds of drop in blood pressure), in which case there is no need to refer
A19.4	**Additional symptoms of anaphylactic shock:** widespread inflammatory response with: • warm extremities • puffy skin and face • difficulty breathing	In anaphylactic shock, the drop in blood pressure is a result of an extreme allergic reaction. In this case, the collapse may be preceded by a patchy swelling of the skin (hives) and worsening asthma. This is an emergency situation, as the symptoms can worsen rapidly to a state of respiratory and circulatory collapse	***

A20: RED FLAGS OF LEUKAEMIA AND LYMPHOMA

TABLE A20 Red flags of leukaemia and lymphoma

Red flag	Description	Reasoning	Priority
A20.1	**Features of bone marrow failure:** symptoms of: • progressive anaemia (see **A18.1**) • recurrent progressive infections • progressive easy bruising, purpura (see **A1.4**) and bleeding	The bone marrow contains the stem cells for the three major cellular components of the blood (red cells, platelets and white blood cells) Bone marrow can fail to produce healthy blood cells if infiltrated by cancer, damaged by medication (including cancer chemotherapy) or radiation, and sometimes as a result of an autoimmune disease Bone marrow failure is a life-threatening situation	***/**
A20.2	**Multiple enlarged lymph nodes** (>1 cm in diameter), but painless, with no other obvious cause (e.g. known glandular fever infection) for more than 2 weeks	Groups of lymph nodes can be found in the cervical region, in the armpits (axillary nodes) and in the inguinal creases (groin). In health, the lymph nodes are usually impalpable masses of soft tissue, but they can enlarge and become more palpable when active in fighting an infection or if infiltrated by tumour cells. If a number of nodes are enlarged (>1 cm in diameter), this may signify a generalised infectious disease such as glandular fever The other important cause of widespread lymph node enlargement (lymphadenopathy) is cancer, and in particular the cancers of the white blood cells (leukaemia and lymphoma) If multiple enlarged lymph nodes are found, it is best to refer for a diagnosis, and as a high priority if the patient is unwell	**/*
A20.3	**A single markedly enlarged lymph node** (>2 cm in diameter) with no other obvious cause	Even in the situation of infection, it is unusual for a lymph node to become grossly enlarged. Cancerous infiltration can lead to a firm, enlarged lymph node, which may be painless. This is particularly typical of lymphoma Unexplained fever, weight loss and itching are other symptoms which, together with lymph node enlargement, are suggestive of lymphoma	**/*

A21: RED FLAGS OF RAISED INTRACRANIAL PRESSURE

TABLE A21 Red flags of raised intracranial pressure

Red flag	Description	Reasoning	Priority
A21.1	**Features of a rapid increase in intracranial pressure:** a rapid deterioration of consciousness leading to coma. Irregular breathing patterns and pinpoint pupils are a very serious sign	An increase in the pressure within the skull seriously threatens the integrity of the structure of the brain. If the pressure increases rapidly (usually as a result of a sudden intracranial haemorrhage or bleeding from a fractured skull), there can follow downwards pressure via the soft tissue of the brain onto the brainstem. The brainstem is the seat of the basic vital functions such as breathing and maintenance of consciousness. As the brainstem is compressed, the patient can lose consciousness, and eventually will stop breathing. Constriction of the pupils is a result of compression of the nerve that leaves the brain at the level of the brainstem to supply the internal muscles of the eye. This is a grave warning sign of impending serious brain damage. Ensure that the patient is in a safe and warm place and, ideally, in the recovery position (unless neck trauma suspected) while waiting for help to arrive	***
A21.2	**Features of a slow increase in intracranial pressure:** progressive headaches and vomiting over the timescale of a few weeks to months. The headaches are worse in the morning and the vomiting may be effortless. Blurring of vision may be an additional symptom	Intracranial pressure will slowly increase if there is a gradual development of a space-occupying lesion, such as a brain tumour, abscess in the brain or accumulation of poorly draining cerebrospinal fluid. The pressure will be worse when the patient has been lying down, and so the symptoms are characteristically worse in the morning. These include blurring of vision, effortless vomiting (i.e. not much preceding nausea) and headache	**

A22: RED FLAGS OF BRAIN HAEMORRHAGE, STROKE AND BRAIN TUMOUR

TABLE A22 Red flags of brain haemorrhage, stroke and brain tumour

Red flag	Description	Reasoning	Priority
A22.1	**Progressive decline in mental and social functioning:** increasing difficulty in intellectual function, memory, concentration and use of language	Gradual loss of mental function can result from a range of slowly developing brain disorders, including dementia, recurrent small strokes, extradural haemorrhage and a slow-growing brain tumour In the elderly in particular, depression can manifest in this way, and the symptoms may resolve with antidepressant medication	*
A22.2	**A temporary loss of neurological function** (usually <2 hours), such as: • loss of consciousness • loss of vision • unsteadiness • confusion • loss of memory • loss of sensation • limb weakness	A temporary loss of neurological function is most commonly seen as part of the syndrome of migraine, in which case it is usually part of a pattern with which the patient is familiar. In migraine, the blood flow to a portion of the brain is temporarily reduced as a result of spasm of an artery. A simple migraine does not merit referral The most common cause of loss of consciousness is a simple faint. This benign syndrome does not merit referral. It is characterised by a low blood pressure and slow but regular pulse, and is triggered by prolonged standing, stuffy conditions and/or emotional arousal. A person who has fainted should start to recover almost immediately after the collapse If these sorts of symptoms occur for the first time, and are not obviously due to a faint or migraine, it is important to exclude the more serious syndrome of transient ischaemic attack (TIA), in which a branch of a cerebral artery has been blocked by the temporary lodging of a small blood clot. A TIA is a warning sign of the more permanent damage that results from stroke, and the patient needs referral as a high priority for diagnosis and treatment If the loss of neurological function has occurred within the past 24 hours and is proving to persist for more than 2 hours (a possible stroke), then referral should be urgent (see **A22.3**).	***/**

TABLE A22 Continued

Red flag	Description	Reasoning	Priority
A22.3	**A persisting loss of neurological function**, such as: • loss of consciousness • loss of vision • unsteadiness • confusion • loss of memory • loss of sensation • muscle weakness	Any development of symptoms that suggest a persisting loss in neurological function merits referral to exclude stroke or a rapidly growing brain tumour Some of these symptoms can also result from disease of the spinal cord (e.g. multiple sclerosis) or of a peripheral nerve (e.g. Bell's palsy). Refer urgently if the loss of neurological function has occurred within the past few hours	***/**
A22.4	**A loss of neurological function that is progressive over the course of days to weeks:** this is more suggestive of a brain tumour than a stroke	(See **A22.3**.) Progressive symptoms of loss of neurological function are more suggestive of brain tumour or degenerative disease (e.g. motor neurone disease) than stroke. However, multiple small strokes can present in this way	**
A22.5	**Features of a slow increase in intracranial pressure:** progressive headaches and vomiting over the timescale of a few weeks to months. The headaches are worse in the morning and the vomiting may be effortless. Blurring of vision may be an additional symptom	Intracranial pressure will slowly increase if there is a gradual development of a space-occupying lesion, such as a brain tumour, abscess in the brain, extradural haemorrhage or accumulation of poorly draining cerebrospinal fluid The pressure will be worse when the patient has been lying down, and so the symptoms are characteristically worse in the morning. These include blurring of vision, effortless vomiting (i.e. not much preceding nausea) and headache	**
A22.6	**Features of a rapid increase in intracranial pressure:** a rapid deterioration of consciousness leading to coma. Irregular breathing patterns and pinpoint pupils are a very serious sign	An increase in the pressure within the skull seriously threatens the integrity of the structure of the brain If the pressure increases rapidly (usually as a result of a sudden intracranial haemorrhage or bleeding from a fractured skull), there can follow downwards pressure via the soft tissue of the brain onto the brainstem. The brainstem is the seat of the basic vital functions, such as breathing and maintenance of consciousness. As the brainstem is compressed, the patient can lose consciousness, and eventually will stop breathing. Constriction of the pupils is a result of compression of the nerve that leaves the brain at the level of the brainstem to supply the internal muscles of the eye. This is a grave warning sign of serious brain damage	***

A23: RED FLAGS OF HEADACHE

TABLE A23 Red flags of headache

Red flag	Description	Reasoning	Priority
A23.1	**Features of a slow increase in intracranial pressure:** progressive headaches and vomiting over the timescale of a few weeks to months. The headaches are worse in the morning and the vomiting may be effortless. Blurring of vision may be an additional symptom	Intracranial pressure will slowly increase if there is a gradual development of a space-occupying lesion, such as a brain tumour, abscess in the brain, extradural haemorrhage or accumulation of poorly draining cerebrospinal fluid. The pressure will be worse when the patient has been lying down, and so the symptoms are characteristically worse in the morning. These include blurring of vision (especially after coughing or leaning forward), effortless vomiting (i.e. not much preceding nausea) and headache	**
A23.2	**A sudden, very severe headache that comes on out of the blue:** the patient needs to lie down and may vomit. There may be neck stiffness (reluctance to move the head) and dislike of bright light	The sudden, very severe headache (like a hit to the back of the head) is a cardinal symptom of the potentially devastating subarachnoid haemorrhage. This is a bleed from an area of weakness in one of the arterial branches that course around the base of the brain (the circle of Willis). Subarachnoid haemorrhage may result from an inherited malformation, and so may develop out of the blue in a seemingly fit person	***
A23.3	**A severe headache that develops over the course of a few hours to days with fever, together with either vomiting or neck stiffness.** The patient may become drowsy or unconscious. Suggests acute meningitis or encephalitis	Meningitis and encephalitis are infections (of the meninges and brain tissue, respectively) that can be caused by a wide range of infectious organisms Although headache and fever are common co-symptoms in benign infections such as tonsillitis, the triad of headache, vomiting and fever is more suggestive of brain infections, and needs to be treated with caution Additional symptoms, such as reluctance to move the head, arching back of the neck and dislike of bright lights, may also be present, and if so are sinister signs. There may be a purpuric rash (see **A23.4**), but the absence of a rash does not rule out the diagnosis	***

TABLE A23 Continued

Red flag	Description	Reasoning	Priority
A23.4	**A severe headache that develops over the course of a few hours to days, with fever and with a bruising and non-blanching rash.** The patient may become drowsy or unconscious. Suggests meningococcal meningitis	(See **A23.3**.) In the form of meningitis caused by *Meningococcus* there can be a serious form of pus-producing infection of the meninges. This carries a risk of septicaemia (multiplying bacteria in the bloodstream) and endotoxic shock (see **A19.3**) Also characteristic of meningococcal septicaemia is the development of an irregularly distributed purpuric rash (like a scattering of pinpoint and larger bruises). The spots in this sort of rash do not blanche (go pale) when pressed, unlike the spots in inflammatory rashes such as the rash of measles This is an emergency situation	***
A23.5	**A severe, one-sided headache over the temple occurring for the first time in an elderly person**	One-sided headaches are common and usually benign, but an unusual, severe, persistent one-sided headache in an elderly person should be taken seriously, as this could reflect the inflammatory condition of temporal arteritis. Temporal arteritis is a form of vasculitis In this condition, inflammation of the arteries supplying the head can become inflamed and thickened, and this carries the risk of obstruction by blood clot There is a significant risk of thrombosis of a cerebral (brain) artery or retinal artery in temporal arteritis, and this is minimised by treatment with corticosteroid medication. Temporal arteritis is more likely to develop in people who have also been diagnosed to have polymyalgia rheumatica (see **A28.3**)	**/***
A23.6	**A long history of worsening (progressive) headaches, with generalised symptoms such as fever, loss of appetite and exhaustion**	Recurrent headaches are common and are usually benign. They are often categorised by doctors as either migraine or tension headaches Consider referral if there is a progression in severity of the headaches, or if there are other symptoms not usually associated with benign headache, such as fever, loss of appetite, weight loss or other neurological symptoms. Benign headaches should respond significantly to treatment, so also consider referral of recurrent headaches if there is no improvement within 1–2 months	*/**

A24: RED FLAGS OF DEMENTIA, EPILEPSY AND OTHER DISORDERS OF THE CENTRAL NERVOUS SYSTEM

TABLE A24 Red flags of dementia, epilepsy and other disorders of the central nervous system

Red flag	Description	Reasoning	Priority
A24.1	**Progressive decline in mental and social functioning:** increasing difficulty in intellectual function, memory, concentration and use of language	Gradual loss of mental function could result from a range of slowly developing brain disorders, including dementia, recurrent small strokes, extradural haemorrhage and a slow-growing brain tumour In the elderly in particular, depression can manifest in this way, and the symptoms may resolve with antidepressant medication	*
A24.2	**Recent onset of confusion** (i.e. evidence of an acute organic mental health disorder): features may include: • confusion • agitation • visual hallucinations • loss of ability to care for self	Organic mental health disorders are, by definition, those that have a medically recognised physical cause, such as drug intoxication, brain damage or dementia Organic disorders are characterised by confusion or clouding of consciousness, and loss of insight. Visual hallucinations may be apparent, as in the case of delirium tremens (alcohol withdrawal) Referral has to be considered if it is recognized that the patient or other people are at serious risk of harm if their condition is not disclosed. As it may be very difficult to fully assess this risk, it is advised that, unless there is absolute confidence that the patient is safe, they should be referred to professionals who are experienced in the treatment of mental health disorders Referral in such a situation may result in the serious outcome of the patient being detained against their will in hospital under a section of the Mental Health Act. As this may be a situation in which patient confidentiality may need to be breached, it is advisable, if there is the time to do so, to seek guidance from your professional body about how to proceed	***/**

TABLE A24 Continued

Red flag	Description	Reasoning	Priority
A24.3	**A temporary loss of neurological function** (usually <2 hours): features may include: • loss of consciousness • loss of vision • unsteadiness • confusion • loss of memory • loss of sensation • limb weakness	A temporary loss of neurological function is most commonly seen as part of the syndrome of migraine, in which case it usually is part of a pattern with which the patient is familiar. In migraine, the blood flow to a portion of the brain is temporarily reduced as a result of spasm of an artery. A simple migraine does not merit referral The most common cause of loss of consciousness is a simple faint. This benign syndrome does not merit referral. It is characterised by a low blood pressure and a slow but regular pulse, and is triggered by prolonged standing, stuffy conditions and/or emotional arousal. A person who has fainted should start to recover almost immediately after the collapse If these symptoms occur for the first time, it is important to exclude the more serious syndrome of transient ischaemic attack (TIA), in which a branch of a cerebral artery has been blocked by the temporary lodging of a small blood clot. A TIA is a warning sign of the more permanent damage that results from stroke, and the patient needs to be referred as a high priority for diagnosis and treatment	**
A24.4	**A persisting loss of neurological function** (lasting >2 hours): features may include: • loss of vision • unsteadiness • confusion • loss of memory • loss of sensation • muscle weakness	Any development of symptoms that suggest a persisting loss in neurological function merits referral to exclude stroke or a rapidly growing brain tumour Some of these symptoms can also result from disease of the spinal cord (e.g. multiple sclerosis) or of a peripheral nerve (e.g. Bell's palsy)	**

TABLE A24 Continued

Red flag	Description	Reasoning	Priority
A24.5	**A first-ever epileptic seizure:** • Generalised tonic–clonic seizure: convulsions, loss of consciousness, bitten tongue, emptying of bladder and/or bowels. This is an emergency if the fit does not settle down within 2 minutes • Generalised absence or complex partial seizures: defined periods of vagueness or loss of awareness, or mood or personality changes • Focal simple seizures: episodes of coarse twitching of one part of the body	Epilepsy most commonly first presents in childhood, and is more common in children who have experienced febrile convulsions. Early diagnosis is important so that early management can help prevent deleterious effects on education and social development. However, it can present at any stage in life, and anyone who may have experienced a first epileptic seizure needs to be referred for diagnosis and advice about driving and personal safety If the seizure occurs during sleep, the only symptom a patient might experience might be a sensation of grogginess in the morning and possibly a wet bed if the bladder has been voided. In such a case, the patient will have no memory of the episode of urination Absence and complex partial seizures may also be difficult to recognise, but are important to refer if suspected, as there is real risk of harm if an episode occurs when performing a risky activity such as climbing or driving A first epileptic seizure may, rarely, result from a brain tumour If a tonic–clonic seizure is ongoing, and particularly if it has lasted for >1 minute, it could develop into an emergency situation, and help needs to be summoned with urgency. It is important to ensure the fitting patient is in the recovery position while help arrives The patient who has experienced a possible seizure must be urged strongly not to drive until they have received medical advice	** If fit is ongoing ***
A24.6	**Progressive coarse tremor appearing in middle to late life**	A fine, symmetrical tremor that is worse with anxiety and overarousal is common and benign, particularly in the elderly In contrast, Parkinson's disease presents with a progressive tremor that is far more coarse and characteristically causes the movement of repeated opposition of thumb and fingers (the so-called 'pill-rolling tremor'). Combined with this there will be increased stiffness of the muscles (the arms will be felt to resist passive movement). Parkinson's disease commonly affects one side more than another in its early stages Commonly, treatment is delayed for as long as is reasonable in Parkinson's disease, so there is no need for high priority referral	*

A25: RED FLAGS OF DISEASES OF THE SPINAL CORD AND PERIPHERAL NERVES

TABLE A25 Red flags of diseases of the spinal cord and peripheral nerves

Red flag	Description	Reasoning	Priority
A25.1	**Any sudden or gradual onset of objectively quantifiable muscle weakness** (e.g. weak grip or difficulty in standing from sitting) For Bell's palsy (facial muscle weakness), see **A25.2**	It is important to distinguish true muscle weakness from a perception of muscle weakness (a common complaint, particularly in people who are depressed). In true muscle weakness there will be real limitation in performing simple day-to-day activities such as brushing the teeth or walking Asking the patient to move muscles against resistance is a simple way of gauging the muscle strength, and is particularly effective in demonstrating if the weakness is asymmetrical (e.g. a one-sided weakness of grip would be very clearly felt on resisted moves of the hands and arms) Muscle weakness may result from conditions of the brain, spinal cord, peripheral nerves and neuromuscular junction, as well as the muscles themselves. As so many of these conditions are potentially serious, it is wise to refer all patients with muscle weakness for a medical diagnosis The rare condition of Guillain–Barré syndrome can lead to a rapidly progressive weakness of the limbs. This would be accompanied by numbness of the hands and feet (it is a peripheral neuropathy). If the patient with these symptoms becomes unable to walk, refer urgently, as the condition, rarely, can progress to affect the respiratory muscles	**/*

TABLE A25 Continued

Red flag	Description	Reasoning	Priority
A25.2	**Bell's palsy (facial weakness)**	Bell's palsy is thought to be the result of a viral infection affecting the facial nerve. In rare cases it may be the result of a more serious underlying condition, such as tumour, multiple sclerosis or Lyme disease The onset can be dramatic, with one-sided facial paralysis developing over the course of 1–2 days The patient may be unable to move the mouth, lift the eyebrows and, importantly, not be able to close the eye on the affected side Bell's palsy requires high priority referral, as early treatment with antiviral and corticosteroid medication may improve the chances of full resolution of symptoms. Also, the health of the cornea of the eye needs to be assessed regularly in the early stages (it can become damaged if the eyelid is not able to be closed fully)	**
A25.3	**Features of polymyalgia rheumatica:** prolonged pain and stiffness and weakness of the muscles of the hips and shoulders associated with malaise and depression Refer urgently if there is a sudden onset of a severe, one-sided temporal headache or visual disturbances	Polymyalgia rheumatica is an inflammatory condition of the muscles of the shoulders and hips, which predominantly afflicts people >50 years old. Because it is inflammatory in nature, there may be associated malaise, but the main symptoms are pain and weakness of the shoulder and hip muscles. Difficulty in standing from a sitting position is a classic sign of hip weakness In polymyalgia rheumatica there is an increased risk of the serious condition of temporal arteritis. Referral is needed for treatment with corticosteroids (see **A23.5**)	* If one-sided headache or visual disturbances are present: ***

TABLE A25 Continued

Red flag	Description	Reasoning	Priority
A25.4	**Any sudden or gradual onset of unexplained, measurable numbness or pins and needles** (either generalised or localised) unless symptoms suggest benign nerve root impingement	Numbness can arise from problems in the brain, spinal cord and the peripheral nerves. All these have potentially serious underlying causes, so if the cause is unclear the patient should be referred for a medical diagnosis Vague numbness is a subjective complaint which is commonly described, but when tested the person can actually distinguish between different types of touch on the 'numb' area. 'Measurable numbness' here refers to the finding that there is the inability to distinguish between the pain of a pin prick and the touch of a piece of cotton wool The most common cause of measurable numbness, however, is compression of nerve roots, in either the neck or sacral region, as a result of osteoarthritis of the spine and sacrum or increased muscle spasm These are benign causes of numbness, and are distinguished by having a one-sided distribution on either the side of an arm and hand or down the back of the leg (sciatica) In this case, if the diagnosis of nerve root impingement is correct, physical treatment (e.g. with acupuncture and massage and specific muscle-stretching exercises) should relieve the numbness as the muscle tension resolves. Refer if there is no improvement in 1 week and urgently if there are any features of cauda equina syndrome (see **A25.5**)	**/*
A25.5	**Cauda equina syndrome:** • numbness of the buttocks and perineum (saddle anaesthesia) • bilateral numbness or sciatica in the legs • difficulty in urination or defecation • impaired sexual function	The cauda equina (horse's tail) is the bunch of nerves that descends from the bottom of the spinal cord from the level of L1–L2 downwards. These nerve roots supply sensation and motor impulses to the perineum, buttocks, groin and legs Cauda equina syndrome suggests the compression of a number of these roots (usually from a central prolapsed disc, but possibly from tumour or other spinal growth). This is a serious situation, as prolonged compression of the perineal nerve supply can lead to permanent problems with urination, defecation and sexual function Refer as a high priority	**

TABLE A25 Continued

Red flag	Description	Reasoning	Priority
A25.6	**The features of early shingles:** intense, one-sided pain, with an overlying rash of crops of fluid-filled reddened and crusting blisters. The pain and rash correspond in location to a neurological dermatome. The pain may precede the rash by 1–2 days	Shingles is an outbreak of the chickenpox virus (varicella zoster) which has lain dormant within a spinal nerve root since an earlier episode of chickenpox. It tends to reactivate when the person is run down, exposed to intense sunlight and is more common in the elderly Warn the patient that the condition is contagious, and advise that immediate treatment (within 48 hours of onset of the rash) with the antiviral drug aciclovir has been proven to reduce the severity of prolonged pain after recovery of the rash. For this reason it is necessary to refer as a high priority to a doctor for advice on medical management	**
A25.7	**Trigeminal neuralgia** (and other forms of one-sided facial pain): lancinating pain on one side of the face, which radiates out from a focal point in response to defined triggers. May be associated with twitching (tic douloureux)	Trigeminal neuralgia is excruciating facial pain, often triggered by light touch or wind, which radiates from a defined point in a predictable distribution on one side of the face The common (and benign) form may be the result of pressure on the trigeminal nerve within the skull by a blood vessel, but rarely is the result of something more serious, such as a brain tumour or multiple sclerosis For this reason, a person with unexplained facial pain should be referred for full investigation Microsurgical treatments have recently been found to have success in intractable cases.	*

A26: RED FLAGS OF DISEASES OF THE BONES

TABLE A26 Red flags of diseases of the bones

Red flag	Description	Reasoning	Priority
A26.1	**Bone pain:** pain originating from bone is characteristically fixed and deep. It may have either an aching or a boring quality. Tenderness on palpation and on percussion (weighty tapping, with the fingertip, of the skin overlying the bone) indicates a structural abnormality such as a fracture. Boring central back pain at night suggests that the origin is the bones rather than muscles. This symptom might suggest bone cancer	It is worth referring any severe or persistent pain that you believe to be originating from bone, as this may originate from an infective, cancerous or degenerative condition of the bone. Possible causes of bone pain include traumatic bruising or fracture, osteomyelitis (bone infection), tumour, Paget's disease, osteoporosis and osteomalacia. The collapse of vertebrae in osteoporosis can lead to a sudden onset of vertebral pain and radiated pain around the front of the body along the line of the affected spinal nerve. Although not usually serious in itself, an osteoporotic collapse needs to be referred for consideration of medical management of the osteoporosis and exclusion of weakening of the bones due to cancer deposits, as this can mimic osteoporosis	**/*

A27: RED FLAGS OF LOCALISED DISEASES OF THE JOINTS, LIGAMENTS AND MUSCLES

TABLE A27 Red flags of localised diseases of the joints, ligaments and muscles

Red flag	Description	Reasoning	Priority
A27.1	**Features of traumatic injury to a muscle or joint:** • sudden onset of pain or swelling in a joint suggesting possible bleeding into the joint (haemarthrosis) • sudden severe pain and swelling around a joint with reluctance to move (sprain or strain, or possible fracture) • sudden onset of tender swelling in a muscle (possible haematoma) • locking of the knee joint (meniscal cartilage tear)	If there are any of these features of traumatic injury to a muscle or joint, it is wise to refer for appropriate immediate assessment (including X-ray imaging) and orthopaedic management. The rest/ice/compression/elevation (RICE) formula should be considered if there is significant inflammation (redness and swelling). 'Rest' means ensuring that the injured region is immobilised, and this needs to be effected by means of recognised first-aid approaches (e.g. splints, bandages, slings)	**

TABLE A27 Continued

Red flag	Description	Reasoning	Priority
A27.2	**Features of intervertebral disc prolapse and severe nerve root irritation:** sudden onset of low back pain so severe that walking is impossible (severe sciatica); difficulty urinating or defecating	In most cases, disc prolapse is not an emergency condition, and may do very well with appropriate complementary medical and massage techniques. Even with sciatic pain it might be expected that appropriate use of many physical therapies might bring relief without need for referral In most cases, the referred pain and weakness indicate compression of one or more of the L3, L4, L5 or S1 nerve roots, and the symptoms are usually one-sided. Expect at least partial relief of these symptoms within a few days of treatment However, medical treatment (anti-inflammatory and muscle relaxant medication) can be very useful if the pain is very severe and there is a lot of muscle spasm, which is not responding to physical therapies Difficulty in urination or defecation or sacral numbness are rare but serious signs which indicate compression of the delicate lower sacral roots (cauda equina syndrome). If these symptoms are apparent, refer for assessment as a high priority (see **A27.3**)	**
A27.3	**Cauda equina syndrome:** • numbness of the buttocks and perineum (saddle anaesthesia) • bilateral numbness or sciatica in the legs • difficulty in urination or defecation • impaired sexual function	The cauda equina (horse's tail) is the bunch of nerves that descends from the bottom of the spinal cord from the level of L1–L2 downwards. These nerve roots supply sensation and motor impulses to the perineum, buttocks, groin and legs Cauda equina syndrome suggests the compression of a number of these roots (usually from a central prolapsed disc, but possibly from tumour or other spinal growth). This is a serious situation, as prolonged compression of the perineal nerve supply can lead to permanent problems with urination, defecation and sexual function Refer as a high priority	**

TABLE A27 Continued

Red flag	Description	Reasoning	Priority
A27.4	**Features of septic or crystal arthritis:** a single, hot, swollen and very tender joint. Patient is unwell. Not usually associated with injury, but may occasionally be caused by a penetrating injury of the joint space	A hot, swollen joint is a sign of possible joint infection. This presents a grave risk to the health of the joint, and needs to be referred so that infection can be excluded However, the most common cause of a single, hot and swollen joint is gout (crystal arthritis), which may respond well to complementary medicine alone. If this is the case, the doctor may wish to prescribe anti-inflammatory medication, but after diagnosis has been confirmed it is worth using simple complementary treatments in the first instance and reserving medication if no improvement is apparent within 3–7 days	**
A27.5	**Unexplained, intense, persistent shoulder pain unrelated to shoulder movement** (for >2 weeks)	Shoulder pain that seems to be unrelated to shoulder movement might be referred from a tumour at the apex of the lung (Pancoast tumour). The common (and benign) causes of shoulder pain include frozen shoulder, shoulder impingement syndrome and acromioclavicular joint inflammation. All are characterised by pain or weakness when attempting to use the affected shoulder. Refer any case in which the pain is not improving with treatment or in which the pain is unrelated to movement	*

A28: RED FLAGS OF GENERALISED DISEASES OF THE JOINTS, LIGAMENTS AND MUSCLES

TABLE A28 Red flags of generalised diseases of the joints, ligaments and muscles

Red flag	Description	Reasoning	Priority
A28.1	**Features of a degenerative arthritis which may benefit from joint replacement:** severe disability from long-standing pain and stiffness in the hips, knees or shoulders	Complementary medical treatment such as acupuncture and osteopathy can be very helpful supportive treatment in advanced osteoarthritis of the hip, knee or shoulder. Referral needs to be considered if the condition is deteriorating to a point at which the activities of daily living are becoming compromised. Refer relatively early, as the patient may need to be put on a waiting list, meaning that surgical treatment may only come after a delay of some weeks to months	*
A28.2	**Any features of an inflammatory arthritis:** symmetrical pain, stiffness and swelling of the joints, or symmetrical stiffness and pain in the sacroiliac joint. May be associated with a fever or sense of malaise	All episodes of inflammatory arthritis (distinguished from osteoarthritis by fairly rapid onset (over days to weeks rather then months to years), joint swelling, fever and general malaise) are best investigated by a conventional practitioner so that autoimmune disease or other serious underlying disease can be excluded. Some forms of inflammatory arthritis are erosive, and powerful medical approaches should be considered to prevent progression and permanent joint damage	**/*
A28.3	**Features of polymyalgia rheumatica:** prolonged pain and stiffness and weakness of the muscles of the hips and shoulders associated with malaise and depression. Refer urgently if there is a sudden onset of a severe, one-sided, temporal headache or visual disturbances	Polymyalgia rheumatica is an inflammatory condition of the muscles of the shoulders and hips which predominantly afflicts people over the age of 50 years. Because it is inflammatory in nature, there may be associated malaise, but the main symptoms are pain and weakness of the shoulder and hip muscles. Difficulty in standing from a sitting position is a classic sign of hip weakness There is an increased risk of the serious condition of temporal arteritis (see **A23.5**). Referral is advised so that the patient can be offered the medical treatment of corticosteroids	**/* If severe, one-sided headache or visual disturbances: ***

A29: RED FLAGS OF DISEASES OF THE KIDNEYS

TABLE A29 Red flags of diseases of the kidneys

Red flag	Description	Reasoning	Priority
A29.1	**Blood in the urine:** • refer all cases in men • refer in women, except in the case of acute urinary infection	The most common and benign cause of blood in the urine in women is bladder infection (cystitis). If the symptoms are suggestive of this diagnosis (burning on urination, low abdominal pain, cloudy or blood-stained urine), there is no need to refer straight away. Treat with complementary medicine, recommend a high fluid intake, and refer only if symptoms are not settling within 3 days However, blood in the urine is not normal in men, who should be protected from infection by the relatively long male urethra Refer all cases of blood in the urine in men, and in women if there are either no other symptoms (blood may be coming from the kidney or from a tumour) or if the pain is felt also in the loin (suggesting a spread of infection to kidneys)	*/**
A29.2	**Unexplained oedema** (excess tissue fluid, manifesting primarily as ankle swelling extending to more than 2 cm above the malleoli)	Oedema means excess tissue fluid. It tends to manifest in the lower regions of the body, first appearing as ankle swelling. It can also become apparent as abdominal and scrotal swelling Mild ankle swelling can develop as a result of inactivity and overheating, but should never extend to more than a couple of centimetres above the malleoli (ankle bones) If the oedema is severe, it may affect the lower part of the calf and can also accumulate in the scrotum, buttocks and lower abdominal tissue If the oedema is due to excess tissue fluid, it will tend to 'pit', meaning that sustained pressure will leave an indentation in the skin Oedema can have a range of causes, and most of these, including kidney disease and chronic heart failure (see **A14.1**), are potentially serious. If the patient is accumulating significant oedema (more than mild ankle swelling), they should be referred for investigation of the cause	**

TABLE A29 Continued

Red flag	Description	Reasoning	Priority
A29.3	**Acute loin pain:** often comes in waves; patient may vomit and collapse	This is characteristic of an obstructed kidney stone. The pain may radiate round to the suprapubic region, particularly if the stone moves some way down the ureter. Encourage drinking of fluids and refer urgently	***
A29.4	**Persistent loin pain** (i.e. pain in the flanks either side of the spine between the levels of T11 and L3)	Persistent achy pain in one or both loins might be an indication of kidney infection or other kidney disease. It would be wise to refer if there is no obvious muscular explanation. Refer as high priority if coexistent with symptoms of cystitis (see **A29.1**) or generalised infection (e.g. fever and malaise)	**
A29.5	**Features of acute pyelonephritis** (kidney infection): fever, malaise, loin pain and cloudy urine suggest an infection of the kidneys	While bladder infections are usually self-limiting, particularly in women, the situation is more serious if there are features indicating that the infection has ascended the ureters to affect the kidney. Acute pyelonephritis carries a risk of permanent scarring of the kidneys, and merits prompt medical attention (treatment with antibiotics)	**
A29.6	**Features of vesicoureteric reflux disease (VUR) in a child:** any history of recurrent episodes or a current episode of cloudy urine or burning on urination should be taken seriously in a pre-pubescent child	Urine infections are common in young children, but need to be taken seriously, particularly if there is a history of recurrent infections. The small child is more vulnerable to VUR, which means that when the bladder contracts, some urine is flushed back towards the kidneys. In the case of infection of the bladder, VUR can lead to infectious organisms causing damage to the delicate structure of the kidney. Sometimes this damage occurs with very few symptoms, but if cumulative and undetected can lead to serious kidney problems and high blood pressure in later life. For this reason, it is wise to refer all pre-pubescent children with a history of symptoms of urinary infections to exclude the possibility of VUR	If no symptoms: * If current symptoms: **
A29.7	**Hypertension of any level with established kidney disease**	Always refer for medical management, as blood pressure should be maintained below 130/80 mmHg in people with kidney disease. There is a much greater risk of worsening kidney damage in patients with hypertension	**/*

A30: RED FLAGS OF DISEASES OF THE URETERS, BLADDER AND URETHRA

TABLE A30 Red flags of diseases of the ureters, bladder and urethra

Red flag	Description	Reasoning	Priority
A30.1	**Acute loin pain:** often comes in waves; patient may vomit and collapse	This is characteristic of an obstructed kidney stone. The pain may radiate around to the suprapubic region, particularly if the stone moves some way down the ureter. Encourage drinking of fluids and refer urgently	***
A30.2	**Blood in the urine (haematuria) or sperm (haemospermia):** • refer all cases in men • refer in women except in the case of acute urinary infection	The most common and benign cause of blood in the urine in women is bladder infection (cystitis). If the symptoms are suggestive of this diagnosis (burning on urination, low abdominal pain, cloudy or blood-stained urine), there is no need to refer straight away. Treat with complementary medicine, recommend a high fluid intake and refer only if symptoms are not settling within 3 days However, blood in the urine is not normal in men, who should be protected from infection by the relatively long male urethra Refer all cases of blood in the urine in men, and in women if there are either no other symptoms (blood may be coming from the kidney or from a tumour) or if the pain is felt also in the loin (suggesting spread of infection to the kidneys) Haemospermia is alarming to the patient but usually benign, as it can result from slight trauma to the genitals. Nevertheless, refer non-urgently to exclude a serious cause	**/*
A30.3	**Features of recurrent or persistent urinary tract infection:** episodes of symptoms including some or all of cloudy urine, burning on urination, abdominal discomfort, blood in urine and fever, especially if occurring in men	Urinary tract infections are generally self-limiting and should clear up within 5 days. Refer anyone who has persistent symptoms in order to exclude an underlying disorder of the urinary system. Recurrent or persistent infections are particularly uncommon in men, and are more likely to signify an underlying disorder of the urinary tract than when they occur in women	**/*

TABLE A30 Continued

Red flag	Description	Reasoning	Priority
A30.4	**Features of a urinary tract infection in a patient in one of the following vulnerable groups:** • pre-existing disorder of the urinary system • diabetes • pregnancy • paraplegia	Refer a patient who develops symptoms of a urinary tract infection straight away for treatment if there is an underlying vulnerability such as known disease of the urinary system (e.g. kidney disease, kidney stones, bladder cancer, enlarged prostate gland), diabetes or pregnancy or if the ability to sense and void the bladder is impaired because of paraplegia In both pregnancy and diabetes, there is a far higher risk of the infection ascending the ureters and damaging the kidneys In pregnancy, urinary tract infections may also increase the risk of early labour or miscarriage	**
A30.5	**Features of moderate prostatic obstruction:** enlargement of the prostate gland leads to symptoms such as increasing difficulty urinating and the need to get up at night to urinate (nocturia)	Benign prostatic enlargement is common, and the symptoms may respond to complementary medical treatment such as western herbs or acupuncture. However, the same symptoms can be caused by a prostatic tumour, and so it is wise to refer for further investigations, including physical (rectal) examination, kidney function tests and a blood test for prostate-specific antigen (PSA)	*
A30.6	**Features of acute pyelonephritis** (kidney infection): fever, malaise, loin pain and cloudy urine suggest an infection of the kidneys	While bladder infections are usually self-limiting, particularly in women, the situation is more serious if there are features indicating that the infection has ascended the ureters to affect the kidney. Acute pyelonephritis carries a risk of permanent scarring of the kidneys, and merits medical attention (treatment with antibiotics)	**
A30.7	**Features of vesicoureteric reflux disease (VUR) in a child:** any history of recurrent episodes or a current episode of cloudy urine or burning on urination should be taken seriously in a pre-pubescent child	Urine infections are common in young children, but need to be taken seriously, particularly if there is a history of recurrent infections. The small child is more vulnerable to VUR, which means that when the bladder contracts, some urine is flushed back towards the kidneys. In the case of infection of the bladder, VUR can lead to infectious organisms causing damage to the delicate structure of the kidney. Sometimes this damage occurs with very few symptoms, but if cumulative and undetected can lead to serious kidney problems and high blood pressure in later life For this reason, it is wise to refer all pre-pubescent children with a history of symptoms of urinary infections to exclude the possibility of VUR	If no symptoms * If current symptoms **

TABLE A30 Continued

Red flag	Description	Reasoning	Priority
A30.8	**Bedwetting in a child:** if persisting over the age of 5 years	Consider referral if the child is over 5 years of age, so that physical causes can be excluded and parents can have access to expert advice	*
A30.9	**Incontinence:** if unexplained or causing distress	A mild degree of stress incontinence (leakage of a small amount of urine when coughing or laughing) is common and benign in women, particularly after childbirth and the menopause. However, uncontrollable losses of large amounts of urine are not normal, nor is bedwetting when asleep. In these cases, investigations are merited to look for treatable causes (e.g. a prolapsed uterus, prostatic obstruction and nocturnal seizures). Also refer so that the patient can have access to guidance and support from an incontinence specialist nurse	*

A31: RED FLAGS OF DISEASES OF THE THYROID GLAND

TABLE A31 Red flags of diseases of the thyroid gland

Red flag	Description	Reasoning	Priority
A31.1	**Goitre:** refer only if symptoms of hyperthyroidism or hypothyroidism are present (see **31.2** and **31.3**), or if the goitre is tender, irregular or noticeably enlarging	A goitre is an enlarged thyroid gland. It can be felt and seen in the lower half of the neck, where it tends to fill the hollow that lies over the trachea and above the manubrium. A small, symmetrical goitre is a not uncommon finding in women, particularly in puberty and pregnancy, and if no symptoms are associated, need not in itself be a cause for referral	*

TABLE A31 Continued

Red flag	Description	Reasoning	Priority
A31.2	**Features of hypothyroidism** (symptoms and signs tend to be progressive over the course of a few months). Symptoms: • tiredness • depression • weight gain • heavy periods • constipation • cold intolerance Signs: • dry puffy skin • dry and thin hair • slow pulse	The symptoms of hypothyroidism (underactive thyroid gland) overlap with those of depression, but a simple blood test can differentiate between the two syndromes If prolonged, the state of hypothyroidism can have significant deleterious metabolic consequences, and medical replacement therapy is advised if it is not responding to complementary medical treatment	*
A31.3	**Features of hyperthyroidism** (these tend to be progressive over the course of a few months). Symptoms: • irritability • anxiety • sleeplessness • increased appetite • loose stools • weight loss • scanty periods • heat intolerance Signs: • sweaty skin • tremor of the hands • staring eyes • rapid pulse	The symptoms of hyperthyroidism overlap with those of an anxiety disorder, but a simple blood test can differentiate between the two syndromes If prolonged, hyperthyroidism can have a significant impact on the cardiovascular system, and medical treatment is advised if not responding to complementary medical treatment High priority referral may be indicated if the patient is very agitated, or if cardiac symptoms (chest pain, palpitations or breathlessness) are present	**/*

Symptoms		Signs
Tiredness		Mental slowness
Loss of appetite		Dementia
Weight gain		Dry thin hair and skin
Cold intolerance		Puffy eyes
Depression		Obesity
Poor libido		Hypertension
Joint and muscle aches		Hypothermia
Constipation		Bradycardia
Heavy periods		Cold peripheries
Psychosis		Oedema
Confusion		Deep voice
		Goitre
		Anaemia

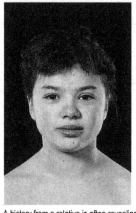

A history from a relative is often revealing
Symptoms of other autoimmune disease
may be present

Figure 2.5 Symptoms and signs of hypothyroidism (see A31.2). (From CTG Figure 5.1c-I.)

Symptoms		Signs
Weight loss		Tremor
Increased appetite		Restlessness
Restlessness		Sweating
Muscle weakness		Irritability
Tremor		Tachycardia
Palpitations		Warm peripheries
Thirst		Exophthalmos
Diarrhoea		Goitre
Scanty periods		
Loss of libido		
Sweating		

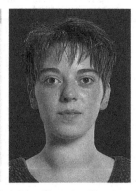

Figure 2.6 The symptoms and signs of hyperthyroidism (see A31.3). (From CTG Figure 5.1c-II.)

A32: RED FLAGS OF DIABETES MELLITUS

TABLE A32 Red flags of diabetes mellitus

Red flag	Description	Reasoning	Priority
A32.1	**Confusion/coma with dehydration** (hyperglycaemia)	Confusion and coma are serious symptoms of uncontrolled diabetes (when the levels of glucose in the blood become too high) and are urgent red flags in their own right If there is any uncertainty whether the cause of the confusion is due to hyperglycaemia or hypoglycaemia, it is wise to administer glucose if the patient is able to take this, or glucagon (by injection) if the patient possesses this treatment. These measures will do no harm if the cause is hyperglycaemia, but can be life-saving if the cause is hypoglycaemia If the patient is losing consciousness, ensure they are kept in a safe place in the recovery position until help arrives	***
A32.2	**Hypoglycaemia** (due to effects of insulin or antidiabetic medication in excess of bodily requirements): agitation, sweating, dilated pupils confusion and coma	Confusion/coma can also be the consequence of a hypoglycaemic attack (a result of an excessive reaction to insulin or antidiabetic medication). This can be helped by urgent administration of glucose in a readily absorbable form (e.g. a glucose drink) or glucagon (by injection) if the patient possesses this treatment If in doubt about the cause of the confusion in a diabetic patient, it is always appropriate to give glucose, as it is safe to do this whatever the cause If the patient is losing consciousness, ensure they are kept in a safe place in the recovery position until help arrives	***
A32.3	**Poorly controlled type 1 or type 2 diabetes:** short history of thirst, weight loss and excessive urination, which is rapidly progressive in severity	Thirst and excessive urination are due to the osmotic effect of glucose in the urine Weight loss occurs because the tissues are unable to utilise the glucose in the situation of a lack of insulin The patient is at high risk of coma because of rising levels of lactic acid Refer as a high priority, and urgently if there are any signs of clouding of consciousness	***/**

TABLE A32 Continued

Red flag	Description	Reasoning	Priority
A32.4	**Untreated type 2 diabetes:** general feeling of unwellness, with thirst and increased need to pass large amounts of urine, which develop over the course of weeks to months	In type 2 diabetes, the onset is more gradual and the situation is less urgent. Sustained levels of hyperglycaemia put the patient at increased risk of heart disease, kidney disease, vascular disease and chronic infections	**/*
A32.5	**Increased tendency to infections such as cystitis, boils and oral thrush (candidiasis)**	Increased tendency to purulent, urinary and skin infections may indicate underlying type 2 diabetes. Any infections in diabetes merit high priority referral for consideration of treatment	*/**
A32.6	**Poor wound healing, especially in the feet and legs**	Increased tendency to poor wound healing may indicate underlying type 2 diabetes. Any poorly healing wounds in diabetes merit high priority referral for consideration of treatment	**/*
A32.7	**Hypertension of any level in diabetes**	Always refer for medical management. Medical guidelines advise that blood pressure should be maintained below 130/80 mmHg in people with diabetes because of the much greater risk of vascular and renal complications which can result from high blood pressure	**/*

A33: RED FLAGS OF OTHER ENDOCRINE DISEASE

TABLE A33 Red flags of other endocrine disease

Red flag	Description	Reasoning	Priority
A33.1	**Features of Cushing's syndrome:** • weight gain • hypertension • weakness and wasting of limb muscles • stretch marks and bruises • mood changes • red cheeks and acne	Cushing's syndrome is due to chronically raised levels of corticosteroids, and may result from excessive bodily production or from medical treatment. It carries serious health consequences in terms of increasing the risk of high blood pressure, diabetes and osteoporosis. Refer if the cause is unknown	*

TABLE A33 Continued

Red flag	Description	Reasoning	Priority
A33.2	**Features of Addison's disease:** • increased skin pigmentation • weight loss • muscle wasting • tiredness • loss of libido • low blood pressure • diarrhoea and vomiting • confusion • collapse with dehydration	Addison's disease is due to a lack of bodily corticosteroid, and the symptoms may develop gradually or may result in a sudden collapse. The syndrome can also result from a sudden withdrawal from high doses of prescribed corticosteroid In both cases, the situation is a medical emergency	***/**
A33.3	**Features of the growth of a pituitary tumour:** progressive headaches, visual disturbance and double vision	The pituitary gland is situated at the base of the brain in the region of the crossing of the optic nerves and the passage of the cranial nerve which supplies the eye muscle A tumour of the pituitary gland may cause early visual disturbance and double vision It can also cause the syndrome of hypopituitarism (see **A33.4**)	**/*
A33.4	**Features of hypopituitarism:** • loss of libido • infertility • menstrual disturbances • tiredness • low blood pressure • inappropriate lactation	The pituitary gland is the source of the endocrine hormones, which regulate growth, metabolism and the reproductive system. Damage to the pituitary gland can result in a complicated pattern of endocrine disturbance. If the cause is a pituitary tumour then the tumour bulk can also cause characteristic problems (see **A33.3**)	**/*
A33.5	**Features of hyperprolactinaemia:** inappropriate secretion of milk and infertility	Prolactin may be secreted in excess in all forms of pituitary disease, and so inappropriate secretion of breast milk is a red flag of a pituitary tumour However, in most cases, inappropriate secretion of milk has a benign cause, or may be the response to medications such as the contraceptive pill	*
A33.6	**Features of acromegaly** (growth hormone excess): • change in facial appearance (coarsening of features) • increased size of hands and feet • enlarging tongue • deepening voice • joint pains • hypertension • breathlessness	Acromegaly commonly results from a pituitary tumour, and so symptoms of pituitary tumour growth (see **A33.3**) may also be present	**/*

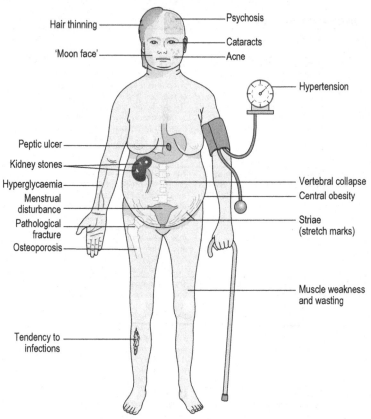

Figure 2.7 The features of Cushing's syndrome (See A33.1). (From CTG Figure 2.2c-l.)

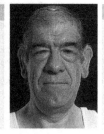

Symptoms	Signs
Change in facial appearance, enlarged hands, feet and hat size, headaches, poor vision, excessive sweating, tiredness, scanty periods, deep voice	Coarse facial features, and thick greasy skin. Lower jaw projects further than upper jaw, gaps between teeth, spade-like hands and feet, hypertension, oedema, weakness of muscles, glucose in the urine

Figure 2.8 The symptoms and signs of acromegaly (see A33.6). (From CTG Figure 5.1e-III.)

A34: RED FLAGS OF MENSTRUATION

TABLE A34 Red flags of menstruation

Red flag	Description	Reasoning	Priority
A34.1	**Primary amenorrhoea:** onset of periods delayed until after age 16 years	Refer any girl for investigation who has not achieved first menstruation by age 16 years	*
A34.2	**Secondary amenorrhoea:** for >6 months	Refer if there have been no periods for 6 months	*
A34.3	**Menorrhagia:** with features of severe anaemia (tiredness, breathlessness, palpitations on exertion)	Menorrhagia (heavy periods) can be the sole cause of significant anaemia, and merits prompt referral for investigation and treatment of the cause. Menorrhagia may result from fibroids, endometriosis or an ovarian cyst	**
A34.4	**Metrorrhagia:** bleeding between periods which has no regular pattern. This includes post-coital bleeding (bleeding after intercourse)	Irregular periods are common, but bleeding that seems to fall outside the normal confines of a 2–5-day menstrual bleed might, rarely, signify a uterine or cervical tumour. In younger women, unexpected bleeding is more likely to signify a sexually transmitted disease, most commonly chlamydia. Breakthrough bleeding is common in women on the contraceptive pill, but this usually falls into a regular pattern. Refer for further investigation if this happens on more than two occasions	*
A34.5	**Post-menopausal bleeding:** any unexplained bleeding after the menopause	Predictable bleeding after the menopause is normal with hormone replacement therapy. Otherwise, any episode of post-menopausal bleeding is a red flag for uterine or cervical tumour. Other causes include uterine polyps	**/*
A34.6	**Vaginal discharge:** after menopause	Vaginal discharge is not normal after the menopause, particularly if offensive or blood-stained. Refer to exclude infection or carcinoma	*

TABLE A34 Continued

Red flag	Description	Reasoning	Priority
A34.7	**Vaginal discharge: before puberty**	Vaginal discharge is not normal before puberty, particularly if offensive or blood-stained. However, the cause is usually benign overgrowth of yeasts or bacteria. Rarely it may be a marker of abuse. Always refer for medical advice (see **A40.34**)	**
A34.8	**Vaginal discharge: in fertile years**	It is normal for there to be a cyclical production of a non-offensive creamy vaginal discharge which peaks in volume around the time of ovulation If the discharge becomes offensive or itchy then this may be a sign of bacterial or yeast overgrowth and could indicate a sexually transmitted infection A patient with unusual discharge can be referred for a free-of-charge confidential consultation to the local genitourinary medicine (GUM) clinic, or to the GP for more tests (see **A35.1**)	*
A34.9	**Vaginal itch (if prolonged)**	Vaginal itch is a common side-effect of thrush (candidiasis) and sensitivity to soaps and bath products, so refer only if prolonged for >1 week and not responding to advice and simple treatment Consider the possibility of atrophic vaginitis in post-menopausal women. This can respond to hormone creams Also, rarely, itch can develop due to lichen sclerosus and vulval cancer Consider the possibility of abuse in children (see **A40.34**). Always refer children with this symptom for investigation	*

A35: RED FLAGS OF SEXUALLY TRANSMITTED DISEASES

TABLE A35 Red flags of sexually transmitted diseases

Red flag	Description	Reasoning	Priority
A35.1	**Vaginal discharge:** if irregular, blood-stained or unusual odour	A slight, creamy vaginal discharge is usual, and tends to increase and become more elastic around the time of ovulation. An increase in this sort of discharge is normal in pregnancy If an irregular pattern of blood staining, volume, itchiness or odour develops, investigation is merited to exclude sexually transmitted disease (STD). This is of particular importance in pregnancy, as some STDs can threaten the health of the fetus If an STD is suspected, advise the patient to visit the local genitourinary medicine (GUM) department for a free-of-charge confidential consultation in the first instance[1] Thrush (candidiasis) does not necessarily merit referral, as it can subside by means of conservative measures and is not usually considered to be contagious. If recurrent and troublesome, consider referral to investigate a possible underlying cause, such as diabetes or immune deficiency	**/*
A35.2	**Vaginal discharge: after menopause**	Vaginal discharge is not normal after the menopause, particularly if of offensive odour or blood-stained. Refer to exclude infection or carcinoma	*
A35.3	**Vaginal discharge: before puberty**	Vaginal discharge is not normal before puberty, particularly if offensive or blood-stained. However, the cause is usually benign overgrowth of yeasts or bacteria Consider the possibility of abuse in children (see **A40.34**). Always refer children with this symptom for investigation	**
A35.4	**Discharge from penis**	Always refer, as this may indicate a sexually transmitted disease (STD). If an STD is suspected, advise the patient to visit the local genitourinary medicine (GUM) department for a free-of-charge confidential consultation in the first instance[1]	*

TABLE A35 Continued

Red flag	Description	Reasoning	Priority
A35.5	**Sores, warty lumps or ulcers on the vagina or penis**	These are very likely to be manifestations of a sexually transmitted infection such as herpes or genital warts. Rarely, they may be cancer. Refer to the local genitourinary medicine (GUM) department[1] for a free of charge confidential consultation in the first instance for investigation	**/*
A35.6	**Pelvic inflammatory disease (PID) (chronic form):** vaginal discharge, gripy abdominal pain, pain on intercourse, dysmenorrhoea, infertility	Chronic PID poses a threat to fertility and may suggest the person has been infected by a sexually transmitted disease (STD). If an STD is suspected, advise the patient to visit the local genitourinary (GUM) department for a free-of-charge confidential consultation[1] or to the GP if symptoms are causing a lot of distress and merit prompt treatment	**/*
A35.7	**Pelvic inflammatory disease (PID) (acute form):** low abdominal pain with collapse, fever	Acute PID poses a serious risk to fertility. Refer urgently for antibiotic treatment. Acute PID may present as the acute abdomen (see **A6.8**)	***
A35.8	**First outbreak of genital herpes:** a cluster of painful ulcers on penis, vulva or around the anal margin. Associated with a feeling of malaise. Inguinal nodes (groin) may be enlarged and tender	Refer to genitourinary medicine (GUM) department for same day treatment as early oral antiviral medication will reduce the length of the painful symptoms and may also reduce the risk of recurrences of the outbreak	*
A35.9	**Outbreak of genital herpes (see A35.8) in the last trimester of pregnancy**	Refer to GP or midwife for discussion of birth plan, as there is a risk of transmission of herpes virus to the baby during delivery	*
A35.10	**Offensive, fishy, watery discharge (possible bacterial vaginosis) in pregnancy**	Refer for treatment, as bacterial vaginosis leads to an increased risk of early labour and miscarriage	**

[1]If you suspect an STD, it is worth discussing with your patient the issue of attending an appointment at the genitourinary medicine (GUM) clinic, so that a proper diagnosis can be made and advice can be given about safe sex and prevention of spread of the condition. Remind your patient that in the UK such a visit will be held in strict confidence by the clinic, and will not be recorded in his or her GP notes.

A36: RED FLAGS OF STRUCTURAL DISORDERS OF THE REPRODUCTIVE SYSTEM

TABLE A36 Red flags of structural disorders of the reproductive system

Red flag	Description	Reasoning	Priority
A36.1	**Primary amenorrhoea:** after age 16 years	Refer any woman for investigation who has not achieved first menstruation by age 16 years If secondary sexual characteristics are developing normally, this might suggest an imperforate hymen or, rarely, an intersex disorder	*
A36.2	**Menorrhagia:** with features of severe anaemia (tiredness, breathlessness, palpitations on exertion)	Menorrhagia (heavy periods) can be the sole cause of significant anaemia, and merits prompt referral for investigation and treatment of the cause Menorrhagia may result from fibroids, endometriosis or an ovarian cyst	**
A36.3	**Post-menopausal bleeding:** any unexplained bleeding after the menopause	Predictable bleeding after the menopause is normal with hormone replacement therapy Otherwise, it is a red flag of uterine or cervical tumour. Refer for further investigation	**/*
A36.4	**Metrorrhagia:** bleeding between periods which has no regular pattern. This includes post-coital bleeding (bleeding after intercourse)	Irregular periods are common, but bleeding that seems to fall outside the normal confines of a 2–5 day menstrual bleed might, rarely, signify a uterine or cervical tumour In younger women, unexpected bleeding is more likely to signify a sexually transmitted disease, most commonly chlamydia Breakthrough bleeding is common in women on the contraceptive pill, but this usually falls into a regular pattern Refer for further investigation if this happens on more than two occasions	*
A36.5	**Pelvic pain or deep pain during intercourse**	Refer as a high priority if pelvic inflammatory disease is a possibility (see **A35.6** and **A35.7**) Otherwise refer routinely so that investigations into the cause can be arranged (may also be the result of endometriosis, fibroids or ovarian cysts)	**/*
A36.6	**Abdominal swelling:** discrete mass in the suprapubic or inguinal region	Always refer for investigations if a mass is felt (possible fibroids, ovarian cyst, tumour, pregnancy)	*

TABLE A36 Continued

Red flag	Description	Reasoning	Priority
A36.7	**Abdominal swelling:** generalised	Refer if the swelling is diffuse and increasing over days to weeks (possible fluid accumulation from a tumour (ascites)) Other possibilities include multiple fibroids, pregnancy and simple weight gain	*
A36.8	**Vulval itch or vaginal discharge in post-menopausal women**	Vaginal itch is a common side-effect of thrush (candidiasis) and sensitivity to soaps and bath products, so refer only if prolonged for >1 week and not responding to advice and simple treatment Consider the possibility of atrophic vaginitis in post-menopausal women. This can respond to hormone creams Also, rarely, itch can develop due to lichen sclerosus and vulval cancer	*
A36.9	**Lump in vulva**	This is usually benign (Bartholin's or sebaceous cyst), but refer for advice about excision and to exclude vulval carcinoma or warts	*
A36.10	**Lump in testicle/ scrotum**	Most scrotal lumps are benign, especially varicocele (sebaceous cyst), but rarely can be testicular cancer. Refer for further investigation	*
A36.11	**Acute testicular pain:** radiates to groin, scrotum or lower abdomen	Refer any sudden onset of severe testicular pain (radiates to groin, scrotum or lower abdomen). This could signify inflammation of the testicle (orchitis) or a twist of the testicle (torsion). If the pain is very intense (with collapse and vomiting), refer as an emergency	***/**
A36.12	**Chronic dull testicular pain:** radiates to groin, scrotum or lower abdomen	If the testicular pain is more of a long-lived discomfort, this could either be chronic epididymitis or varicocele, and merits a medical examination and further tests	*
A36.13	**Precocious puberty:** secondary sexual characteristics before age 8 years in girls and 9 years in boys	Refer if secondary sexual characteristics begin to appear before age 8 years in girls and 9 years in boys so that an unusual endocrine cause can be excluded	*
A36.14	**Delayed puberty:** secondary sexual characteristics not apparent by age 15 years in girls and 16 years in boys	Refer if secondary sexual characteristics have not started to appear by age 15 years in girls and 16 years in boys. Refer if menstruation has not begun by the time of a girl's 16th birthday (primary amenorrhoea)	*

A37: RED FLAGS OF PREGNANCY

TABLE A37 Red flags of pregnancy

Red flag	Description	Reasoning	Priority
A37.1	**Bleeding:** any episode of vaginal bleeding in pregnancy	Refer all cases to the GP to arrange investigation (ultrasound scan). Slight, painless bleeding occurring at 4, 8, or 12 weeks of gestation is most likely to be physiological (i.e. benign) in nature, but refer to exclude miscarriage Painless or painful bleeding at a later stage in pregnancy may result from placenta praevia or placental abruption, both of which are a serious threat to the health of the fetus and the mother Refer as an emergency if there are any signs of shock (see A19.3), as internal bleeding may not be immediately apparent	***/**
A37.2	**Abdominal pain:** any episode of sustained abdominal pain in pregnancy	Gripy abdominal pains (like mild period pains) are common in early pregnancy, and if they do not prevent daily activities are not worrying Severe or worsening abdominal pain in early pregnancy may be the first indication of ectopic pregnancy, and needs to be referred on the same day Severe pain in later pregnancy may be a symptom of placental abruption, and likewise merits urgent referral. It also can be the first sign of pre-eclampsia Abdominal pain is particularly serious if any signs of shock are apparent (see **A19.3**), as internal bleeding may not be immediately apparent Periodic, mild, cramping sensations in later pregnancy (lasting no more than a few seconds) are likely to be benign Braxton Hicks contractions. If becoming regular and intensifying, these might signify premature labour (if before week 36 of pregnancy) or labour. If in any doubt, refer for an assessment	***
A37.3	**Nausea and vomiting with dehydration** for >1 day in pregnancy	Refer if unremitting (patient unable to drink freely for more than 1 day) or if there are any features of dehydration (see **A3.5**). The patient may need hospital admission for administration of fluids	**

TABLE A37 Continued

Red flag	Description	Reasoning	Priority
A37.4	**Oedema** in pregnancy	Mild swelling of the ankles and hands is common in middle to late pregnancy Refer if oedema extends to >2 cm above the malleoli, if there is facial oedema or if there is an associated rise in blood pressure of >15 mmHg above the usual blood pressure, or any degree of hypertension (systolic >140 mmHg, diastolic >90 mmHg). All these signs suggest the possibility of pre-eclampsia Occasionally, oedema can develop as a result of an undiagnosed cardiac abnormality	✱✱
A37.5	**Palpitations** in pregnancy	Usually, when palpitations are experienced there is the occasional missed beat, and this is nothing to worry about. However, the increased cardiac output may lead to a previously undiagnosed heart abnormality becoming apparent Refer if the pulse rate is either rapid (>100 beats/minute) or irregular, or if there are frequent missed beats (more than 1 every 5 beats) Remember that palpitations may result from the added strain on the cardiovascular system that results from anaemia in pregnancy	✱✱
A37.6	**Pubic symphysis pain** in pregnancy	Refer for a medical assessment of the pain if it is not responding to treatment, and if it is affecting mobility (may benefit from expert physiotherapy advice and aids)	✱✱
A37.7	**Anaemia** (tiredness, depression, breathlessness, palpitations) in pregnancy	Anaemia is common in pregnancy. The risks of bleeding during labour are higher in women with anaemia, so medical wisdom is that if significant it should be treated with iron replacement	✱
A37.8	**Itching (severe), especially of the palms and soles**, in pregnancy	May result from cholestasis, a condition that can damage the fetus. Refer as a high priority so that appropriate blood tests can be performed	✱✱
A37.9	**Potential pregnancy-induced hypertension (PIH)**	Refer if you find that the blood pressure has risen to 30 mmHg systolic or 15 mmHg diastolic above any measurement taken previously	✱
A37.10	**Mild pregnancy-induced hypertension (PIH)**	Refer if the diastolic blood pressure is 90–99 mmHg, and the systolic blood pressure is <140 mmHg	✱

TABLE A37 Continued

Red flag	Description	Reasoning	Priority
A37.11	**Moderate to severe pregnancy-induced hypertension (PIH)**	Refer as a high priority if the diastolic blood pressure is >100 mmHg or the systolic blood pressure is >140 mmHg	**
A37.12	**Features of pre-eclampsia/HELLP syndromes:** • headache • abdominal pain • visual disturbance • nausea and vomiting • oedema (in middle to late pregnancy)	Headache, abdominal pain and visual disturbances can presage eclampsia, even in the absence of raised blood pressure Nausea and vomiting, headache and oedema together suggest the development of the HELLP syndrome (haemolysis, liver abnormalities and low platelets) Both these syndromes, which may overlap, are absolute emergencies	***
A37.13	**Thromboembolism:** pain in the calf, swollen or discoloured leg, or breathlessness, with chest pain or blood in the sputum in pregnancy	Refer any features of a thromboembolic event, i.e. deep venous thrombosis (DVT) of the calf or pelvic veins (see **A11.7**), pulmonary embolus (see **A17.10**) or stroke (see **A22.3**) as an emergency The risks of these events are greater in pregnancy. Thromboembolism is the most significant cause of maternal death in pregnancy	***
A37.14	**Fever:** refer in pregnancy if high (>38.5°C) and no response to treatment in 24 hours	Refer for management of the underlying cause as high fever may affect the embryo/fetus	**
A37.15	**Fever with rash in the first trimester of pregnancy**	Refer suspected rubella or chickenpox so that the health of the embryo/fetus can be monitored	**
A37.16	**Fever with rash in the last trimester of pregnancy**	Refer if chickenpox or shingles is suspected, as there is a risk of fatal fetal varicella infection	**
A37.17	**Outbreak of genital herpes (see A35.8) in the last trimester of pregnancy**	Refer to GP or midwife for discussion of birth plan, as there is a risk of transmission of herpes virus to the baby during delivery	*
A37.18	**Urinary tract infection** in pregnancy	Always refer for urine testing for bacteria as if present there is an increased risk of induction of miscarriage in the first trimester, and also chronic kidney infection in the mother	**
A37.19	**Offensive, fishy smelling discharge** (possible bacterial vaginosis) in pregnancy	Refer for treatment, as bacterial vaginosis leads to an increased risk of early labour and miscarriage	**

TABLE A37 Continued

Red flag	Description	Reasoning	Priority
A37.20	**Any watery vaginal leakage in middle to late pregnancy**	A very watery discharge in middle to late pregnancy is amniotic fluid until proven otherwise. Premature rupture of the membranes (PRM) carries a risk of uterine infection, and needs to be assessed as a high priority. Even if the pregnancy has come to term, PRM without the onset of labour carries this risk, and conventional practice is to induce labour, if has not started naturally, within 24 hours of PRM	**

A38: RED FLAGS OF THE PUERPERIUM (THE 8 WEEKS THAT FOLLOW DELIVERY)

TABLE A38 Red flags of the puerperium (the 8 weeks that follow delivery)

Red flag	Description	Reasoning	Priority
A38.1	**Fever in the puerperium**	Refer any case of fever developing in the first 2 weeks of the puerperium (temperature >38°C for >24 hours) to exclude possible uterine infection	**
A38.2	**Post-partum haemorrhage:** refer if bleeding is any more than a blood-stained discharge	Blood-stained discharge (lochia) is normal in the early puerperium, but moderate to severe bleeding (like a heavy period or heavier) is not, and needs to be referred as it can herald a more serious bleed A profuse bleed of >500 mL or the symptoms of shock (see **A19.3**) constitute an emergency.	***/**
A38.3	**Thromboembolism:** pain in the calf, discoloured or swollen leg, or breathlessness with chest pain or blood in the sputum in the puerperium	Refer any features of a thromboembolic event, i.e. deep venous thrombosis (DVT) of the calf or pelvic veins (see **A11.7**), pulmonary embolus (see **A17.10**) or stroke (see **A22.3**) as an emergency The risks of these events are greater in the puerperium	***
A38.4	**Post-natal depression**	Refer any case of depression developing in the post-natal period, lasting for >3 weeks and not responding to treatment Refer straight away if the woman is experiencing suicidal ideas, or if you believe the health of the baby is at risk	**

TABLE A38 Continued

Red flag	Description	Reasoning	Priority
A38.5	**Post-natal psychosis**	Refer straight away if you suspect the development of post-natal psychosis (delusional or paranoid ideas and hallucinations are key features), as this condition is associated with a high risk of suicide or harm to the baby	**
A38.6	**Insufficient breast milk**	Refer if the mother is considering stopping breastfeeding within the first few months after delivery because of apparently insufficient milk production. In the case of poor latching on of the baby, advice from an expert breastfeeding adviser, midwife or health visitor will often remedy the problem	**/*
A38.7	**Sore nipples/ blocked ducts during the time of breastfeeding**	Refer to the midwife (early days) or health visitor for advice on breastfeeding technique and for treatment of possible thrush infection. Encourage the mother to keep feeding despite the discomfort, as a continued flow of milk can help with healing	**
A38.8	**Mastitis during the time of breastfeeding** not responding to treatment in 2 days	Refer if not responding to treatment within 2 days, or if you suspect the development of an abscess (a firm mass is felt in the affected breast, and the mother feels very unwell). Encourage the mother to keep feeding despite the discomfort, as a continued flow of milk can help with the healing	**/*

A39: RED FLAGS OF DISEASES OF THE BREAST

TABLE A39 Red flags of diseases of the breast

Red flag	Description	Reasoning	Priority
A39.1	**Insufficient breast milk when breastfeeding**	Refer if the mother is considering stopping breastfeeding within the first few months after delivery because of apparently insufficient milk production. In the case of poor latching on of the baby, advice from an expert breastfeeding adviser, midwife or health visitor will often remedy the problem	**/*

TABLE A39 Continued

Red flag	Description	Reasoning	Priority
A39.2	Lactation/nipple discharge but not breastfeeding	The production of milk or nipple discharge in someone who is not breastfeeding or during late pregnancy may be a sign of a pituitary disorder or breast cancer, and investigation is merited (see **A33.5**) However, in most cases, inappropriate secretion of milk has a benign cause, or may be the response to medications such as the contraceptive pill	*
A39.3	Sore nipples/ blocked ducts during the time of breastfeeding	Refer to the midwife (early days) or health visitor for advice on breastfeeding technique and for treatment of possible thrush infection. Encourage the mother to keep feeding despite the discomfort, as a continued flow of milk can help with healing	**
A39.4	Mastitis during the time of breastfeeding not responding to treatment in 2 days	Refer if not responding to treatment within 2 days, or if you suspect the development of an abscess (a firm mass is felt in the affected breast, and the mother feels very unwell). Encourage the mother to keep feeding despite the discomfort, as a continued flow of milk can help with the healing	**/*
A39.5	Inflamed breast tissue but not breastfeeding	Inflammation of a portion of a breast is common in breastfeeding mothers (mastitis), but needs prompt assessment if it occurs in someone who is not lactating, as this may signify inflammation from an underlying tumour	**/*
A39.6	Pain in the breast but no inflammation or lump	Tenderness in the breast tissue is common and usually results from periodic pre-menstrual hormone stimulation. This symptom can be asymmetrical Pain is not a usual symptom of breast cancer, and an anxious patient can be reassured. The patient should be questioned to ensure that the pain is not actually chest pain, because angina can present with pain that may be described as pain in the breast	*
A39.7	Lump in the breast	When a breast lump is found, skin dimpling and fixity or irregularity of the lump are more sinister signs Tender lumps are more likely to be benign cysts Conventional medical practice in the UK is now to refer all suspicious lumps in the breast for prompt assessment, because it is known that 1 in 10 breast lumps are found to be cancerous. For this reason, all cases of breast lumps should be referred to the GP for further investigation	*

TABLE A39 Continued

Red flag	Description	Reasoning	Priority
A39.8	**Breast tissue development in teenage boys and adult men (gynaecomastia)**	Refer any case of gynaecomastia in a teenage boy or adult male. A pubescent boy can be reassured that this problem (if confined to breast-bud development) is a common feature of puberty which should settle down, but refer nevertheless to exclude rare endocrine diseases. Adult men with this condition need investigations to exclude cancerous change and endocrine disorders	*
A39.9	**Eczema of nipple region**	A one-sided, crusty, non-healing skin disorder of the nipple may be a form of cancer (Paget's disease). This particularly affects middle-aged women. Refer for investigation	*

A40: RED FLAGS OF CHILDHOOD DISEASES

TABLE A40 Red flags of childhood diseases

Red flag	Description	Reasoning	Priority
A40.1	**Maternal concern**	Any condition in which the parent is very concerned about the health of the child is worth referring for a second opinion. The parent is the person who will know best if something is not right with the child, even if it is not very specific. It is wise to respect this instinct, as small children sometimes do not generate very specific symptoms even when seriously unwell	**/*
A40.2	**Inconsolable baby:** for >3 hours	Although this feature is very common and usually benign, consider referral if inconsolable and unexplained crying (for at least 3 hours) starts in a previously settled baby	**
A40.3	**Childhood cancer:** red flags include progressive symptoms – loss of weight, sweats, poor appetite, an unexplained lump or mass or an enlarged unilateral lymph node (>1.5 cm in diameter), recurrent infections, bruising, anaemia and bleeding	Refer any case in which there is a short history of unexplained symptoms that have arisen within the past weeks to months and which are progressive. Also, refer as a high priority if there are red flags of bone marrow failure (see **A1.4**)	**/*

TABLE A40 Continued

Red flag	Description	Reasoning	Priority
A40.4	**Any fever in a child <3 months old**	Infections in infants can become serious conditions very quickly because of the immature immune system, poor temperature control and small size. They lead easily to high fever and dehydration. The infant is at increased risk of convulsions and circulatory collapse However, in this age group, fever is common and usually is *not* serious	**
A40.5	**Fever >38.5°C in a child** (<8 years old) if not responding to treatment in 2 hours	High fevers can promote convulsions in young children. Treatment to bring the temperature down includes keeping the environment cool, tepid sponging, gentle alternative treatments such as acupuncture/homeopathy and antipyretic medication such as paracetamol or ibuprofen suspension	**
A40.6	**Febrile convulsion: ongoing**	Refer a case in which the convulsion is not settling within 2 minutes as an emergency. Ensure the child is kept in a safe place and in the recovery position while help arrives	***
A40.7	**Febrile convulsion: recovered**	Refer all cases in which the child has just suffered a febrile convulsion (the parents need advice on how to manage future fits, and the child should be examined by a doctor)	**
A40.8	**Dehydration in an infant** (<3 years old): signs include dry mouth and skin, loss of skin turgor (firmness), drowsiness, sunken fontanelle and dry nappies	A dehydrated infant is at high risk of circulatory collapse because of their small size and immature homeostatic mechanisms. Infants who are dehydrated may lose the desire to drink, and so the condition can rapidly deteriorate	***/**
A40.9	**Dehydration in children (>3 years old) if severe or prolonged for >48 hours:** signs include dry mouth and skin, loss of skin turgor, low blood pressure, dizziness on standing and poor urine output	Although not as unstable as an infant, a dehydrated child or adult still needs hydration to prevent damage to the kidneys. Referral should be made if the patient is unable to take fluids or if the dehydration persists for >48 hours	**

TABLE A40 Continued

Red flag	Description	Reasoning	Priority
A40.10	**Confusion in older children with fever**	Confusion is common and usually benign in young children (<8 years old) when a fever develops. However, it is not usual in older children, who should be referred to exclude central nervous system involvement (e.g. meningitis or brain abscess)	**
A40.11	**Any features of a notifiable disease**[1]	All the immunisable diseases are notifiable diseases. The complementary medical practitioner should consider referral of these cases so that the GP can report the episode to the local Health Protection Agency	**
A40.12	**Vomiting:** refer if persistent, and either a cause of distress to the child (i.e. not possetting), a cause of dehydration or if projectile	Vomiting is common in children, and usually self-limiting. In babies, regurgitation of milk is normal (possetting), and not a cause for concern if the child is contented and continuing to gain weight. Refer if there are features of dehydration, or if the vomiting is projectile (a feature of pyloric stenosis in newborn babies). Food poisoning and infectious bloody diarrhoea are notifiable diseases[1]	**
A40.13	**Diarrhoea:** if persistent, and associated with either dehydration, poor weight gain, weight loss or chronic ill-health	Chronic loose stools in a child may signify the presence of an infectious organism, coeliac disease or inflammatory bowel disease. Refer as a high priority if dehydration is present (see **A40.8** and **A40.9**). Food poisoning and infectious bloody diarrhoea are notifiable diseases[1]	**/*
A40.14	**Soiling with faeces** (in underwear or bed)	Always refer for diagnosis if persistent and appearing in a previously continent child (could signify constipation with faecal overflow, a developmental problem of the bowel or emotional disturbance)	*
A40.15	**Recurrent or constant intense abdominal pain:** if pain is associated with fever, vomiting, collapse, and rigidity and guarding on examination	All these features are signs of the acute abdomen (see **A6.8**), which in children is most commonly due to appendicitis or a form of bowel obstruction (from a twist or obstruction in a hernia). Urgent surgical assessment is required. All these conditions can spontaneously resolve, but a recurrence is likely. Refer for treatment or assessment	***/**

TABLE A40 Continued

Red flag	Description	Reasoning	Priority
A40.16	**Recurrent mild abdominal pain**	Features of abdominal pain in children which suggest a more benign (functional) cause include mild pain which is worse in the morning, location around the umbilicus and pain worse with anxiety. Refer only if the child is not responding to your treatment	*
A40.17	**Jaundice** (yellowish skin, yellow whites of the eyes and possibly dark urine and pale stools)	Jaundice is always of concern in children and babies with the exception of the mild form of jaundice which can affect the newborn. Refer all cases to ensure serious liver disease is excluded	**
A40.18	**Any new onset of difficulty breathing** (i.e. increased respiratory rate,[2] nocturnal wheeze or noisy breathing) in a small child (<8 years old) Also if there is unexplained sudden blockage of one nostril	Always take a new onset of difficulty breathing in a child seriously, and refer for medical assessment to exclude serious disease. Common causes include lower respiratory tract infections, asthma, allergic reactions, inhalation of foreign bodies and congenital heart disease A nostril may suddenly block after the unwitnessed insertion of a foreign body. This is a serious situation, as the foreign body (e.g. a pea) is at risk of becoming inhaled	***/**
A40.19	**Complications of tonsillitis:** severe constitutional upset not responding to treatment within 5 days	Tonsillitis is common and usually self-limiting in children. The child should be back to their usual self within 3–4 days, so refer if there is no improvement after this time period	**
A40.20	**Complications of tonsillitis:** a single grossly enlarged infected tonsil (quinsy) in an unwell and feverish child	Quinsy is the development on an abscess in the tonsil. It carries a serious risk of obstruction of the airways and requires a same-day surgical opinion. Refer urgently if the child is experiencing any restriction in breathing (stridor may be heard) (see **A40.21**)	***/**
A40.21	**Stridor** (harsh noisy breathing heard on both the inbreath and the outbreath)	Stridor is a noise that suggests upper airway obstruction. It is a serious red flag if it develops suddenly. It suggests possible swelling of the air passages due to laryngotracheitis, quinsy or epiglottitis. If restriction to breathing is significant, the patient with stridor will be sitting very still It is important not to ask to see the tongue, as this can affect the position of the epiglottis, and may worsen the obstruction Exposing the patient to steam (from a nearby kettle or running shower) can alleviate swelling while you wait for help to arrive	***/**

TABLE A40 Continued

Red flag	Description	Reasoning	Priority
A40.22	**Features of severe asthma:** at least two of the following: • rapidly worsening breathlessness • increased respiratory rate[2] • reluctance to talk because of breathlessness • need to sit upright and still to assist breathing • cyanosis is a very serious sign (see **A17.12**)	Severe asthma is a potentially life-threatening condition and may develop in someone who has no previous history of severe attacks Urgent referral is required so that medical management of the attack can be instigated Keep the child as calm as possible while you wait for help to arrive 'Cyanosis' describes the blue colouring that appears when the blood is poorly oxygenated. Unlike the blueness from cold, which affects only the extremities, central cyanosis from poor oxygenation can be seen on the tongue	***
A40.23	**Bed wetting:** if persisting over the age of 5 years	Consider referral if the child is >5 years old, so that physical causes can be excluded and the parents can have access to expert advice	*
A40.24	**Features of vesicoureteric reflux disease (VUR) in a child:** any history of recurrent episodes or a current episode of cloudy urine or burning on urination should be taken seriously in a pre-pubescent child	Urine infections are common in young children but need to be taken seriously, particularly if there is a history of recurrent infections. The small child is more vulnerable to VUR, which means that when the bladder contracts, some urine is flushed back towards the kidneys In the case of infection of the bladder, VUR can lead to infectious organisms causing damage to the delicate structure of the kidney. Sometimes this damage occurs with very few symptoms, but if cumulative and undetected can lead to serious kidney problems and high blood pressure in later life For this reason it is wise to refer all pre-pubescent children with a history of symptoms of urinary infections to exclude the possibility of VUR Refer children with current symptoms as a high priority, and those who are currently well non-urgently	*/**

TABLE A40 Continued

Red flag	Description	Reasoning	Priority
A40.25	**Acute testicular pain:** radiates to the groin, scrotum or lower abdomen	Refer any sudden onset of severe testicular pain (radiates to the groin, scrotum or lower abdomen). This could signify inflammation of the testicle (orchitis) or a twist of the testicle (torsion). If the pain is very intense (with collapse and vomiting), refer as emergency	**/***
A40.26	**Precocious puberty:** secondary sexual characteristics appearing before age 8 years in girls and 9 years in boys	Refer if secondary sexual characteristics begin to appear before age 8 years in girls and 9 years in boys so that an endocrine cause can be excluded	*
A40.27	**Delayed puberty:** secondary sexual characteristics not apparent by age 15 years in girls and 16 years in boys	Refer if secondary sexual characteristics have not started to appear by the age of 15 years in girls and 16 years in boys. Refer if menstruation has not begun by the time of a girl's 16th birthday (primary amenorrhoea)	*
A40.28	**Epilepsy:** refer any child who has suffered a suspected blank episode (absence) or seizure (see **A24.5**)	Epilepsy most commonly first presents in childhood, and is more common in children who have experienced febrile convulsions. Early diagnosis is important as early management can help prevent deleterious effects on education and social development.	*
A40.29	**Squint or double vision:** in any child if previously undiagnosed	Refer any child who demonstrates a previously undiagnosed squint. In young children this usually results from a congenital weakness of the external ocular muscles, but needs ophthalmological assessment to prevent long-term inhibition of depth vision. If appearing in an older child it may signify a tumour of the brain, pituitary gland or orbital cavity	*

TABLE A40 Continued

Red flag	Description	Reasoning	Priority
A40.30	**Complications of acute otitis media in a child:** persistent fever/pain/confusion for >3–4 days after the onset of the earache (may indicate spread of the infection, e.g. mastoiditis or brain abscess)	Otitis media is an uncomfortable but self-limiting ear infection which commonly affects young children. It is now considered good practice not to prescribe antibiotics in a simple case, which will generally settle within 1–3 days, sometimes after natural perforation of the eardrum. This is a beneficial healing process (so some sticky discharge for 1–2 days after an earache is not a cause for concern) However, persisting high fever, confusion or intense pain is not usual, and the child should be referred to exclude the rare possibility of infectious complications	**
A40.31	**New onset of difficulty hearing in a child:** lasting for >3 weeks	Refer if prolonged, if interfering with social interactions and education or if associated with pain in the ear or dizziness. The most likely cause is glue ear, a chronic accumulation of mucoid secretions in the middle ear	*
A40.32	**Persistent discharge from the ear in a child**	Chronic discharge from the ear for >1 week after the infection of otitis media has settled down may indicate the development of chronic otitis media, and this needs further investigation as there is risk of permanent damage to the middle ear	*
A40.33	**Features of autism:** • slow development of speech • impaired social interactions • little imaginative play • obsessional repetitive behaviour	Mild degrees of autism may not be diagnosed until the child reaches secondary school age Refer if you are concerned that the child is demonstrating impaired social interactions (aloofness), impaired social communication (very poor eye contact, awkward and inappropriate body language) and impairment of imaginative play (play may instead be dominated by obsessional behaviour such as lining up toys or checking). Early diagnosis can result in the child being offered extra educational and psychological support	*

TABLE A40 Continued

Red flag	Description	Reasoning	Priority
A40.34	**Sexual or physical abuse:** • unexplained or implausible injuries • miserable, withdrawn child • still, watchful child – 'frozen watchfulness' • overtly sexualised behaviour in a pre-pubescent child • vaginal or anal discharge or itch	All the listed features may have a benign explanation, but if you have any concerns you should take the situation very seriously In the UK, you can start by seeking confidential advice from the NSPCC helpline or from the local Safeguarding Board which is the statutory organisation responsible for dealing with child protection. In the UK, the Safeguarding Boards operate from the local county councils Suspected child abuse is a situation in which you might have to break your professional obligation of confidentiality If you have any concerns about doing this, discuss the case with the ethics advisor from your professional body	**

[1]Notifiable diseases: notification of a number of specified infectious diseases is required of doctors in the UK as a statutory duty under the Public Health (Infectious Diseases) 1988 Act and the Public Health (Control of Diseases) 1988 Act and, more recently, the Health Protection (Notification) Regulations 2010. The UK Health Protection Agency (HPA) Centre for Infections collates details of each case of each disease that has been notified. This allows analyses of local and national trends. This is one example of a situation in which there is a legal requirement for a doctor to breach patient confidentiality.

Diseases that are notifiable include: acute encephalitis, acute poliomyelitis, acute infectious hepatitis, anthrax, cholera, diphtheria, enteric fevers (typhoid and paratyphoid) food poisoning, infectious bloody diarrhoea, leprosy, malaria, measles, meningitis (bacterial and viral forms), meningococcal septicaemia (without meningitis), mumps, plague, rabies, rubella, SARS, scarlet fever, smallpox, tetanus, tuberculosis, typhus, viral haemorrhagic fever, whooping cough and yellow fever.

[2]Categorisation of respiratory rate in children

The normal range for respiratory rate in children varies according to age.

The following rates indicate moderate to severe breathlessness:

newborn (0–3 months)	>60 breaths/minute
infant (3 months to 2 years)	>50 breaths/minute
young child (2–8 years)	>40 breaths/minute
older child to adult	>30 breaths/minute

A41: RED FLAGS OF DISEASES OF THE SKIN

TABLE A41 Red flags of diseases of the skin

Red flag	Description	Reasoning	Priority
A41.1	**A rapidly enlarging patch(es) of painful, crusting or swollen red skin**	Crusting, spreading skin disease suggests erysipelas or severe impetigo. If spreading rapidly, antibiotic treatment should be considered Refer with some urgency if this occurs in someone with eczema, as it can rapidly become a serious condition (or it may indicate herpes virus infection of the broken skin)	**
A41.2	**A rapidly advancing region or line of redness tracking up the skin of a limb** (following the pathway of a lymphatic vessel)	This suggests the deep spread of infection from a distal site (cellulitis and/or lymphangitis), and should be considered for antibiotic treatment	**
A41.3	**Pronounced features of candidal infection** (thrush) of the skin or mucous membranes of the mouth	Widespread candidiasis suggests an underlying chronic condition such as immunodeficiency or diabetes mellitus Refer to exclude underlying disease	*
A41.4	**The features of early shingles:** intense, one-sided pain, with an overlying rash of crops of fluid-filled reddened and crusting blisters. The pain and rash correspond in location to a neurological dermatome. The pain may precede the rash by 1–2 days	Shingles is an outbreak of the chickenpox virus (varicella zoster) which has lain dormant within a spinal nerve root since an earlier episode of chickenpox. It tends to reactivate when the person is run down, exposed to intense sunlight and is more common in the elderly Warn the patient that the condition is contagious, and advise that immediate treatment (within 48 hours of onset of the rash) with the antiviral drug aciclovir has been proven to reduce the severity of prolonged pain after recovery of the rash. For this reason it is necessary to refer as a high priority to a doctor for advice on medical management	**
A41.5	**Generalised itch**	Generalised itch (not eczema) suggests an underlying medical cause (e.g. cholestasis), iron deficiency or cancer. It may also result from scabies. Refer for diagnosis if persisting over a few days	*
A41.6	**Itching (severe),** especially of the palms and soles, in pregnancy	May result from cholestasis, a condition that can damage the fetus. Refer as a high priority	**

TABLE A41 Continued

Red flag	Description	Reasoning	Priority
A41.7	**Large areas of redness affecting most (>90%) of the body surface (erythroderma):** refer because of the risk of dehydration and loss of essential salts	Erythroderma can develop in severe cases of eczema and psoriasis and as a reaction to some medications. It can become a medical emergency, as the cardiovascular system can become under strain from the massively increased blood flow to the skin that results from the generalized inflammation	***/**
A41.8	**Generalised macular rash** (flat, red spots)	Refer if you suspect the possibility of a notifiable disease (i.e. rubella, measles or scarlet fever)[1] NB: Chickenpox is not a notifiable disease, and there is no need to refer if there are no other red flags. A patient with chickenpox needs to be advised about the risk of contagiousness which is significant within the first 5 days of developing the rash	*/**
A41.9	**Purpura or bruising rash** (non-blanching)	A rash that contains areas of non-blanching or bruising suggests a bleeding disorder or vasculitis. Refer as an emergency if the patient is also acutely unwell with headache/fever or vomiting (possible meningococcal infection; see **A23.4**)	***/**
A41.10	**Any lumps/moles with features suggestive of malignancy:** • recent change in shape • irregularity • a tendency to bleed • crusting • >5 mm in diameter • irregularities in pigmentation • intense black colour	Skin tumours include basal-cell carcinomas, squamous-cell carcinomas and malignant melanomas Pre-malignant skin tumours are often associated with changes due to sun damage (on the scalp, temples and the backs of the hands), and appear as spreading, flat areas of dark pigmentation, or irregular scabs that never seem to heal Seborrhoeic keratoses are benign waxy darkened warty growths found on ageing skin which are no need for concern, but may be confused with tumours If you have any doubt it is worth referring for an early diagnosis	*
A41.11	**Progressive swelling of the soft tissues of the face and neck (angio-oedema) and/ or urticaria (nettle rash)**	Angio-oedema can result from an acute allergic reaction and can precede life-threatening asthma. Refer urgently if there are any features of respiratory distress (itchy throat/wheeze)	***

TABLE A41 Continued

Red flag	Description	Reasoning	Priority
A41.12	**Hirsutism** (unexplained hairiness)	Refer any unexplained increase in body hair in middle life, as this may indicate an endocrine disease or, in women, polycystic ovary syndrome	*

[1]Notifiable diseases: notification of a number of specified infectious diseases is required of doctors as a statutory duty under the UK Public Health (Infectious Diseases) 1988 Act and the Public Health (Control of Diseases) 1988 Act. The UK Health Protection Agency (HPA) Centre for Infections collates details of each case of each disease that has been notified. This allows analyses of local and national trends. This is one example of a situation in which there is a legal requirement for a doctor to breach patient confidentiality.

Diseases that are notifiable include: acute encephalitis, acute poliomyelitis, anthrax, cholera, diphtheria, dysentery, food poisoning, leptospirosis, malaria, measles, meningitis (bacterial and viral forms), meningococcal septicaemia (without meningitis), mumps, ophthalmia neonatorum, paratyphoid fever, plague, rabies, relapsing fever, rubella, scarlet fever, smallpox, tetanus, tuberculosis, typhoid fever, typhus fever, viral haemorrhagic fever, viral hepatitis (including hepatitis A, B and C), whooping cough and yellow fever.

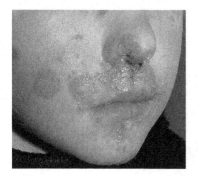

Figure 2.9 The crusting rash of impetigo (see A41.1). (From CTG Figure 5.4d-VI.)

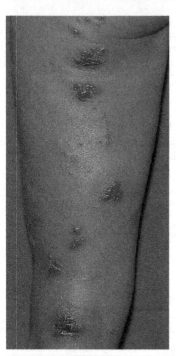

Figure 2.10 Shingles on the back of the leg (see A41.4). (From CTG Figure 5.4d-IV.)

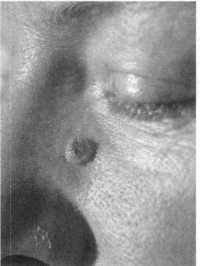

Figure 2.11 A malignant but slow growing basal cell carcinoma on the cheek (see A41.10). (From CTG Figure 6.1c-XIX.)

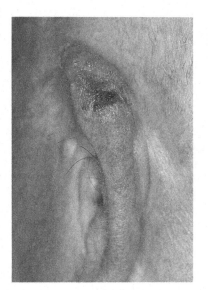

Figure 2.12 A malignant but slow growing squamous cell carcinoma on the earlobe (see A41.10). (From CTG Figure 6.1c.)

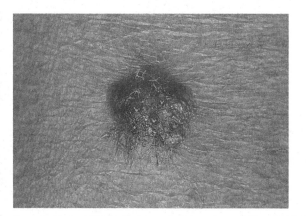

Figure 2.13 A malignant skin tumour (nodular melanoma) (see A41.10). (From Kumar and Clark, 6th edn, Figure 23.34.)

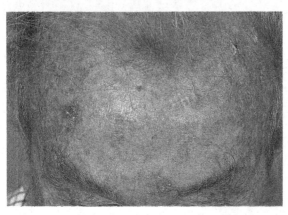

Figure 2.14 Pre-malignant solar keratoses on the sun-exposed forehead (see A41.10). (From CTG Figure 6.1c-XVIII.)

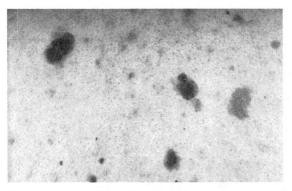

Figure 2.15 Benign seborrhoeic warts on the skin of the back (see A41.10). (From CTG Figure 6.1c-XVI.)

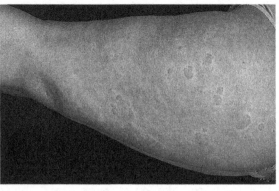

Figure 2.16 Wheals on the arm in urticaria, one of the features of angio-oedema (see A41.11). (From CTG Figure 6.1c-XXIII.)

A42: RED FLAGS OF DISEASES OF THE EYE

TABLE A42 Red flags of diseases of the eye

Red flag	Description	Reasoning	Priority
A42.1	**An intensely painful and red eye**	A painful red eye could result from iritis, choroiditis, acute glaucoma, corneal ulcer or keratitis. All these are serious conditions, and the patient should be advised to attend either their GP or the nearest eye emergency department for early assessment	***/**
A42.2	**A painful, red and swollen eye and eyelids:** patient (often a child) is very unwell	If the eye and the surrounding tissues are intensely painful and swollen, this could be a spreading infection of the soft tissues of the eye (orbital cellulitis). Refer urgently to the emergency department	***
A42.3	**A painful eye with no obvious inflammation:** eye movements are painful	Deep, intense pain exacerbated by eye movement is characteristic of optic neuritis or choroiditis. Refer as a high priority to the nearest emergency department	**

TABLE A42 Continued

Red flag	Description	Reasoning	Priority
A42.4	**Discharge from the eye:** if severe, prolonged and painful, or if seen in the following vulnerable groups: • the newborn • immunocompromised • malnourished	Discharge from the eye(s) is usually the result of acute allergic, bacterial or viral conjunctivitis, and as such is usually self-limiting, and will not necessarily require antibiotic treatment. Advise the patient that he or she may be very contagious while the eye is discharging Only consider referral if the discharge continues for >5 days or if there is any pain	**
A42.5	**Sudden onset of painless blurring or loss of sight in one or both eyes**	Loss of sight or blurring in one or both eyes may be due to thromboembolic disease, optic neuritis, retinal tear or corneal ulcer. Some of these conditions require high priority treatment to prevent blindness, so refer as a high priority to nearest emergency department When floaters and blurring occur out of the blue in middle age these are usually the result of the benign condition of vitreous detachment. Nevertheless, referral is advised to exclude the more serious possible causes	***/**
A42.6	**Sudden onset of painless blurring or loss of sight in one or both eyes accompanied by one-sided headache**	Loss of sight accompanied by a headache in an older person (>50 years) may represent temporal arteritis. This is more likely to occur in someone who has been diagnosed with polymyalgia rheumatica (see **A28.3**). Urgent treatment with corticosteroids may prevent progression to blindness. Refer urgently to the nearest emergency department	***/**
A42.7	**Gradual onset of painless blurring or loss of sight in one or both eyes**	Refer for assessment, as treatment of the causes of gradual loss of sight may prevent progressive deterioration of the sight Causes include refractive error, cataract, glaucoma and macular degeneration	*

TABLE A42 Continued

Red flag	Description	Reasoning	Priority
A42.8	**Squint:** in any child if previously undiagnosed	Refer any child who demonstrates a previously undiagnosed squint. In young children, this usually results from a congenital weakness of the external ocular muscles, but needs ophthalmological assessment to prevent long-term inhibition of depth vision. If appearing in older children, it may signify a tumour of the brain, pituitary or orbital cavity	*
A42.9	**Recent onset of double vision in an adult**	Double vision suggests a physical distortion of the orbital cavity or damage to a cranial nerve. Refer as a high priority	**
A42.10	**Recent onset of drooping eyelid (ptosis)**	Ptosis suggests damage to a nerve due to a tumour, or muscle wasting disease. Refer for investigation	*
A42.11	**Features of thyroid eye disease:** staring eyes, whites visible above and below pupils, inflamed conjunctivae, symptoms of hyperthyroidism (tremor, agitation, weight loss, palpitations)	Thyroid eye disease results from specific antibodies that are generated in Graves' disease. If severe it can threaten the health of the eyes, as soft tissue builds up in the orbit, pushing the eye forward and putting pressure on the optic nerve	*
A42.12	**Inability to close the eye**	The eye may not close fully in thyroid eye disease and also in Bell's palsy. This can rapidly lead to serious damage to the conjunctiva and cornea (which rely on the moistness of tears to remain healthy) A simple first-aid treatment is to keep the affected eye shut with a pad held in place with medical tape until medical advice has been sought	**
A42.13	**Foreign body in the eye**	If there is a foreign body that cannot be removed, gently keep the lid closed by means of a pad and medical tape and arrange urgent assessment at the nearest eye emergency department	**

A43: RED FLAGS OF DISEASES OF THE EAR

TABLE A43 Red flags of diseases of the ear

Red flag	Description	Reasoning	Priority
A43.1	**Vertigo in a young person:** lasting for >6 weeks, or if so severe as to be causing recurrent vomiting, or if patient may be at increased risk of stroke (e.g. in pregnancy, or previous episode)	The most likely cause of a sudden onset of dizzy spells in a young person is an inflammation of the inner ear (labyrinthitis). This usually settles down completely within 6 weeks. Medical treatment is to prescribe anti-sickness medication, so only refer if the sickness does not respond to your treatment. Rarely, a sudden onset of dizziness is the consequence of a stroke or multiple sclerosis. Consider referral if there has been any previous episode of neurological disturbance (e.g. blurred vision or numbness) or if there is an increased risk or history of thromboembolic disease	**/*
A43.2	**Vertigo in an older person** (>45 years old)	Refer so that the patient can have investigations to exclude the possibility of stroke (dizziness can result from brainstem or cerebellar stroke). See **A22.3**	**/*
A43.3	**Complications of acute otitis media:** persistent fever/pain/ confusion for >3–4 days after the onset of the earache (may indicate spread of the infection, e.g. mastoiditis or brain abscess)	Otitis media is an uncomfortable but self-limiting ear infection which commonly affects young children. It is now considered good practice not to prescribe antibiotics in a simple case, which will generally settle within 1–3 days, sometimes after natural perforation of the eardrum. This is a beneficial healing process (so some sticky discharge for 1–2 days after an earache is not a cause for concern). However, persisting high fever, confusion or intense pain is not usual, and the child should be referred to exclude the rare possibility of infectious complications	**
A43.4	**Persistent discharge from the ear**	Chronic discharge from the ear for >1 week after the infection of otitis media has settled down may indicate the development of chronic otitis media, and this needs further investigation, as there is risk of permanent damage to the middle ear	*

TABLE A43 Continued

Red flag	Description	Reasoning	Priority
A43.5	**Features of mastoiditis:** fever, with a painful and swollen mastoid bone (the bony prominence of the skull immediately behind the ear)	Mastoiditis is a now rare complication of otitis media, and usually affects children. It is a serious condition, as it is a bone infection and so can be difficult to treat with antibiotics Refer as a high priority	**
A43.6	**New onset of difficulty hearing in a child:** lasting for >3 weeks	Refer if prolonged, if interfering with social interactions and education, or if associated with pain in the ear or dizziness. The most likely cause is glue ear, a chronic accumulation of mucoid secretions in the middle ear	*
A43.7	**Sudden onset of absolute deafness** (one-sided or bilateral)	Absolute deafness suggests damage to the acoustic nerve or auditory centres of the brain, and requires high priority assessment	**
A43.8	**Gradual onset of relative deafness in an adult for >7 days**	A degree of hearing loss is common after a cold, but has usually subsided within a week. If hearing loss is slow and progressive, referral for audiometric assessment is advised to exclude the rare, but treatable, slowly growing acoustic neuroma However, the accumulation of earwax is possibly the most common cause of hearing loss in adults. This can be easily excluded by examination of the ear with the otoscope	*
A43.9	**Tinnitus if progressive or if associated with hearing loss**	Tinnitus (ringing or buzzing in the ear) is usually a benign finding, and remains fairly constant, or may increase in times of stress. It is not normally progressive or associated with hearing loss, and if it is, this may suggest a progressive disorder of the ear or the auditory nerve. Refer to the GP for audiometric assessment	*
A43.10	**Earache in an adult for >3 weeks**	Earache is common after a cold, but should subside within a week or so. If persistent (>3 weeks) and unexplained, referral is merited as this is a red flag for cancer of the nasopharynx	*

A44: RED FLAGS OF MENTAL HEALTH DISORDERS

TABLE A44 Red flags of mental health disorders

Red flag	Description	Reasoning	Priority
A44.1	**Suicidal thoughts:** with features that suggest serious risk (old age, male sex, social isolation, concrete plans in place)	This symptom may not be volunteered by a person suffering from depression. A question like 'Have you ever thought life is not worth living?' may reveal suicidal ideation Thoughts that life is not worth living do not necessarily signify serious risk, but if present should lead you to question further about features that suggest seriousness of intent and a high-risk social situation High-risk factors include old age, being a man, isolation or marital separation, and concrete plans in place about how to end it all (e.g. clearly thought out method; stockpiling medications, the writing of notes to those who will be left as a result of the suicide) If you have any concerns that your patient is at a serious risk of suicide, you should urge them to discuss their situation with the GP and to seek treatment for their low mood. You may wish to discuss the situation with the doctor yourself, but should seek the patient's permission before you do this The patient may be resistant to the idea of referral. Only if you have grave concerns that the patient is a risk because of mental illness, or others around them are at risk, does this becomes a situation when it may be appropriate to breach your normal practice of confidentiality. In such circumstances it would be essential to first seek advice from a medico-legal expert such as the professional conduct officer of your professional body	**

TABLE A44 Continued

Red flag	Description	Reasoning	Priority
A44.2	**Hallucinations, delusions or other evidence of thought disorder, together with evidence of deteriorating self-care and personality change**	These are all features of a psychosis such as schizophrenia. Suicide risk is high As it may be very difficult for you to fully assess this risk, it is advised that, unless you are absolutely sure of the patient's safety, you should refer him or her to professionals who are experienced in the treatment of mental health disorders. Ideally you should seek the patient's consent before you speak to a health professional Referral in such a situation may result in the serious outcome of the patient being detained in hospital against their will under a section of the Mental Health Act The patient may be resistant to the idea of referral. Only if you have grave concerns that the patient is a risk because of mental illness, or others around them are at risk, does this becomes a situation when it may be appropriate to breach your normal practice of confidentiality. In such circumstances it would be essential to first seek advice from the professional conduct officer of your professional body.	**
A44.3	**Features of mania:** increasing agitation, grandiosity, pressure of speech and sleeplessness with delusional thinking	Mania is a feature of bipolar disorder, and is a form of psychosis that carries a high risk of behaviour which can be both socially and physically damaging to the patient and to those around them. Suicide risk is high As it may be very difficult for you to fully assess this risk, it is advised that, unless you are absolutely sure of the patient's safety, you should refer him or her to professionals who are experienced in the treatment of mental health disorders. Ideally you should seek the patient's consent before you speak to a health professional Referral in such a situation may result in the serious outcome of the patient being detained in hospital against their will under a section of the Mental Health Act The patient may be resistant to the idea of referral. Only if you have grave concerns that the patient is a risk because of mental illness, or others around them are at risk, does this becomes a situation when it may be appropriate to breach your normal practice of confidentiality. In such circumstances it would be essential to first seek advice from the professional conduct officer of your professional body.	**

TABLE A44 Continued

Red flag	Description	Reasoning	Priority
A44.4	**Evidence of an organic mental health disorder:** e.g. confusion, deterioration in intellectual skills, loss of ability to care for self	Organic mental health disorders are, by definition, those that have a medically recognised physical cause, such as drug intoxication, brain damage or dementia. They are characterised by confusion or clouding of consciousness, and loss of insight. Visual hallucinations may be apparent, as in the case of delirium tremens (alcohol withdrawal) It is advised that, unless you are absolutely sure of the patient's safety, you should refer him or her to professionals who are experienced in the treatment of mental health disorders. Ideally you should seek the patient's consent before you speak to a health professional Referral in such a situation may result in the serious outcome of the patient being detained in hospital against their will under a section of the Mental Health Act The patient may be resistant to the idea of referral. Only if you have grave concerns that the patient is a risk because of mental illness, or others around them are at risk, does this becomes a situation when it may be appropriate to breach your normal practice of confidentiality. In such circumstances it would be essential to first seek advice from the professional conduct officer of your professional body.	✱✱
A44.5	**Severe depression/ obsessive–compulsive disorder or anxiety:** if not responding to treatment and seriously affecting quality of life	In certain cases of minor mental health disorder, the symptoms of depression, obsessive thoughts or anxiety can be so overwhelming as to be disabling. Referral needs to be considered for psychiatric or psychological support if these symptoms appear to be seriously affecting quality of life (e.g. the patient is unable to leave their home)	✱

TABLE A44 Continued

Red flag	Description	Reasoning	Priority
A44.6	**Severe disturbance of body image:** if not responding to your treatment, and resulting in features of progressive anorexia nervosa or bulimia nervosa (e.g. progressive weight loss, secondary amenorrhoea, repeated compulsion to bring about vomiting)	Severe forms of eating disorder can result in progressive ill-health, which can be so severe as to be life-threatening. If symptoms are not responding to your treatment, you should consider referral for professional psychiatric support
The patient may be resistant to the idea of referral. Only if you have grave concerns that the patient is a risk because of mental illness, or others around them are at risk, does this becomes a situation when it may be appropriate to breach your normal practice of confidentiality. In such circumstances it would be essential to first seek advice from the professional conduct officer of your professional body.	*
A44.7	**Features of autism in a child:** • slow development of speech • impaired social interactions • little imaginative play • obsessional repetitive behaviour	Mild degrees of autism may not be diagnosed until the child reaches secondary school age. Refer if you are concerned that the child is demonstrating impaired social interactions (aloofness), impaired social communication (very poor eye contact, awkward and inappropriate body language) and impairment of imaginative play (play may instead be dominated by obsessional behaviour such as lining up toys or checking), as early diagnosis can result in the child being offered extra educational and psychological support	*
A44.8	**Post-natal depression**	Refer any case of depression developing in the post-natal period which is lasting for >3 weeks, and which is not responding to your treatment. Refer straight away if the woman is experiencing suicidal ideas, or if you believe the health of the baby to be at risk
The patient may be resistant to the idea of referral. Only if you have grave concerns that the patient is a risk because of mental illness, or others around them are at risk, does this becomes a situation when it may be appropriate to breach your normal practice of confidentiality. In such circumstances it would be advisable to first seek advice from the professional conduct officer of your professional body.	**/*

TABLE A44 Continued

Red flag	Description	Reasoning	Priority
A44.9	Post-natal psychosis	Refer straightaway if you suspect the development of post-natal psychosis (delusional or paranoid ideas and hallucinations are key features), as this condition is associated with a high risk of suicide or harm to the baby The patient may be resistant to the idea of referral. Only if you have grave concerns that the patient is a risk because of mental illness, or others around them are at risk, does this becomes a situation when it may be appropriate to breach your normal practice of confidentiality. In such circumstances it would be advisable to first seek advice from the professional conduct officer of your professional body.	**

CHAPTER 3

B TABLES: RED FLAGS ORDERED BY SYMPTOM KEYWORD

INTRODUCTION

The B tables present red flags ordered by symptom keyword. In each table the red flags are also prioritised according to urgency so that those meriting the most rapid response are found at the top of the list.

These lists are designed for quick access and summarise information in a very brief way. The reader is in all cases given a reference to lead them to consult the explanations found in the A tables in Chapter 2 for more detailed explanations and definitions of medical terms.

The order of the B tables can be found in the contents pages of this text.

TABLE B1 Red flags of abdominal pain and swelling

Symptoms suggestive of:	Priority	For more detail and definitions go to:
Severe abdominal pain with collapse (the acute abdomen): the pain can be constant or colicky (coming in waves); rigidity, guarding and rebound tenderness are serious signs The acute abdomen can be caused by: • acute pancreatitis: presents as the acute abdomen with severe central abdominal and back pain, vomiting and dehydration • ruptured aortic aneurysm: acute abdominal or back pain with collapse; features of shock (low blood pressure and rapid pulse) may be coexistent • obstructed gallbladder. Right hypochondriac pain (pain under the right ribs) which is very intense and comes in waves. May be associated with fever, vomiting and jaundice	***/**	A6. Red flags of diseases of the stomach A7. Red flags of diseases of the pancreas A9. Red flags of diseases of the gallbladder A10. Red flags of diseases of the small and large intestines A11. Red flags of diseases of the blood vessels
Pelvic inflammatory disease (acute form): low abdominal pain with collapse and fever Offensive vaginal discharge may be an additional feature	***/**	A35. Red flags of sexually transmitted diseases
Acute testicular pain: radiates to groin, scrotum or lower abdomen. May be vomiting and collapse	***/**	A36. Red flags of structural disorders of the reproductive system

TABLE B1 Continued

Symptoms suggestive of:	Priority	For more detail and definitions go to:
Acute loin pain (pain in flanks radiating round to pubic region): comes in waves. May be vomiting, agitation and collapse. Suggests obstructed kidney stone	***/**	A30. Red flags of diseases of the ureters, bladder and urethra
Severe abdominal pain in pregnancy: refer as emergency if any signs of shock are apparent (see **A19.3**) If periodic mild cramping sensations in later pregnancy (lasting no more than a few seconds) are becoming regular and intensifying, these might signify early labour (if before week 36 of pregnancy) or labour	***/**	A37. Red flags of pregnancy
Pre-eclampsia/HELLP syndromes in pregnancy: headache, abdominal pain, visual disturbance, nausea and vomiting and oedema (in middle to late pregnancy)	***	A37. Red flags of pregnancy
Right hypochondriac pain (pain under the right ribs) with malaise for >3 days suggests chronic biliary or hepatic disease	**/*	A8. Red flags of diseases of the liver A9. Red flags of diseases of the gallbladder
Recurrent or persistent urinary tract infection: episodes of symptoms including some or all of cloudy urine, burning on urination, abdominal discomfort, blood in urine and fever, especially if occurring in men. If occurring in women, no need to refer if settling down within 5 days	**/*	A30. Red flags of diseases of the ureters, bladder and urethra
Signs of an inguinal hernia: swelling in groin which is more pronounced on standing, especially if uncomfortable	**/*	A10: Red flags of diseases of the small and large intestines
Pelvic inflammatory disease (chronic form): vaginal discharge, gripy abdominal pain, pain on intercourse, dysmenorrhoea, infertility	**/*	A35. Red flags of sexually transmitted diseases
Pelvic pain or deep pain during intercourse: suggests ovarian or uterine inflammation	**/*	A36. Red flags of structural disorders of the reproductive system
Early shingles: intense, one-sided abdominal pain, with overlying rash of crops of fluid-filled reddened and crusting blisters. The pain may precede the rash by 1–2 days. Refer for early consideration of antiviral treatment	**	A25. Red flags of diseases of the spinal cord and peripheral nerves
Stable aortic aneurysm: pulsatile tubular mass in abdomen >5 cm in diameter. Usually affects people >50 years old, and is associated with the degenerative changes of atherosclerosis	*	A11. Red flags of diseases of the blood vessels

TABLE B1 Continued

Symptoms suggestive of:	Priority	For more detail and definitions go to:
Chronic pancreatitis: central abdominal and back pain, weight loss and loose stools over weeks to months	*	A7. Red flags of diseases of the pancreas
Epigastric pain or dyspepsia: only if for the first time in someone >40 years old or if resistant to treatment after 3 months	*	A6. Red flags of diseases of the stomach
Abdominal swelling: discrete suprapubic or inguinal mass. Possible fibroids, ovarian cyst, tumour, pregnancy	*	A36. Red flags of structural disorders of the reproductive system
Abdominal swelling – generalised and painless: Possible fluid accumulation from a tumour (ascites)	*	A1. Red flags of cancer A36. Red flags of structural disorders of the reproductive system
Chronic dull testicular pain: may radiate to groin, scrotum or lower abdomen. Possible epididymitis or varicocele	*	A36. Red flags of structural disorders of the reproductive system

TABLE B2 Red flags of anaemia

Anaemia is the term describing any state in which the oxygen-carrying ability of the red blood cells is reduced and the concentration of haemoglobin in the blood is lower than normal

Symptoms suggestive of:	Priority	For more detail and definitions go to:
Bone marrow failure: severe progressive anaemia, recurrent progressive infections or bruising, purpura and bleeding	***/**	A1. Red flags of cancer A20. Red flags of leukaemia and lymphoma
Severe anaemia: pallor, extreme tiredness, breathlessness on exertion, feeling of faintness, depression, sore mouth and tongue. Excessive bruising and severe visual disturbances There may also be features of strain on the cardiovascular system: chest pain on exertion, features of tachycardia and increasing oedema	**	A18. Red flags of anaemia
Pernicious anaemia (vitamin B$_{12}$ deficiency): tiredness, lemon-yellow pallor and gradual onset of neurological symptoms (numbness, weakness)	**/*	A18. Red flags of anaemia
Long-standing anaemia: pallor, tiredness, breathlessness on exertion, feeling of faintness, depression, sore mouth and tongue	*	A18. Red flags of anaemia
Anaemia in pregnancy: pallor, tiredness, breathlessness on exertion. The risks of bleeding during labour are higher in women with anaemia, so refer for treatment	*	A37. Red flags of pregnancy

TABLE B3 Red flags of anxiety or agitation

Symptoms suggestive of:	Priority	For more detail and definitions go to:
Hypoglycaemia (due to effects of insulin or antidiabetic medication in excess of bodily requirements): agitation, sweating, dilated pupils, confusion and coma	***	A32. Red flags of diabetes mellitus
Hallucinations, delusions or other evidence of thought disorder together with evidence of deteriorating self-care and personality change. All features of a psychosis such as schizophrenia. Suicide risk is high. Refer urgently if behaviour is posing a risk to the patient or others	***/**	A44. Red flags of mental health disorders
Mania: increasing agitation, grandiosity, pressure of speech and sleeplessness with delusional thinking. All features of bipolar disorder, a form of psychosis, which carries a high risk of behaviour that can be both socially and physically damaging to the patient. Suicide risk is high. Refer urgently if behaviour is posing a risk to the patient or others	***/**	A44. Red flags of mental health disorders
Post-natal psychosis: delusional or paranoid ideas and hallucinations are key features. This condition is associated with a high risk of suicide or harm to the baby. Refer urgently if behaviour is posing a risk to the patient or others	***/**	A38. Red flags of the puerperium
Organic mental health disorder (i.e. due to underlying gross physical abnormality): confusion, agitation, deterioration in intellectual skills, loss of ability to care for self. (Possible organic brain disorder such as drug intoxication, brain damage or dementia)	***/**	A44. Red flags of mental health disorders
Hyperthyroidism: irritability, anxiety, sleeplessness, increased appetite, loose stools, weight loss, scanty periods and heat intolerance. Signs: sweaty skin, tremor of the hands, staring eyes and rapid pulse	**/*	A31. Red flags of diseases of the thyroid gland
Severe depression/obsessive–compulsive disorder or anxiety: if not responding to treatment and seriously affecting quality of life	*	A44. Red flags of mental health disorders
Severe disturbance of body image: resulting in features of progressive anorexia nervosa or bulimia nervosa (e.g. progressive weight loss, secondary amenorrhoea, repeated compulsion to bring about vomiting)	*	A44. Red flags of mental health disorders

TABLE B4 Red flags of bleeding or blood loss

Symptoms suggestive of:	Priority	For more detail and definitions go to:
Severe blood loss leading to shock: if the following symptoms and signs have been present for more than a few minutes (i.e. not just simple faint) or are worsening: dizziness, fainting and confusion. Rapid pulse of >100 beats/minute. Blood pressure <90/50 mmHg. Cold and clammy extremities	***	A19. Red flags of haemorrhage and shock
Bone marrow failure: symptoms of progressive anaemia, recurrent progressive infections, progressive bruising, purpura and bleeding	***/**	A20. Red flags of leukaemia and lymphoma
Vomiting of fresh blood or altered blood (haematemesis): if blood is altered, it looks like dark gravel or coffee grounds in the vomit	***/**	A6. Red flags of diseases of the stomach A8. Red flags of diseases of the liver
Altered blood in stools (melaena): stools look like black tar. Suggests large amount of bleeding from stomach	***/**	A6. Red flags of diseases of the stomach
Any episode of vaginal bleeding in pregnancy: refer as an emergency if any signs of shock are apparent (low blood pressure, fainting, rapid pulse), as internal bleeding may not become immediately apparent. Otherwise refer as a high priority for investigation of cause	***/**	A37. Red flags of pregnancy
Post-partum haemorrhage: if bleeding after childbirth is any more than a blood-stained discharge A profuse bleed of >500 mL or the symptoms of shock (low blood pressure, fainting, rapid pulse rate) constitutes an emergency	***/**	A38. Red flags of the puerperium
Continuing blood loss: any situation in which significant bleeding is continuing for more than a few minutes without any signs of abating (e.g. nosebleed), except within the context of menstruation	***/**	A19. Red flags of haemorrhage and shock
Unexplained bleeding: either from the surface of the skin or emerging from an internal organ, such as the bowel, bladder or uterus	**	A1. Red flags of cancer
Infectious bloody diarrhoea or food poisoning: any episode of diarrhoea and vomiting in which food is suspected as the origin, or in which blood appears in the stools. These are notifiable diseases	**	A10. Red flags of diseases of the small and large intestines
Blood mixed in with stools: fresh blood mixed in with the stools suggests colonic or rectal origin Blood that drips after passage of stools is anal in origin and is usually benign (no need to refer)	**	A10. Red flags of diseases of the small and large intestines

TABLE B4 Continued

Symptoms suggestive of:	Priority	For more detail and definitions go to:
Coughing up of blood (haemoptysis): (if on only a single occasion, only amounts more than a teaspoon in volume are significant)	**	A17. Red flags of lower respiratory disease
Tuberculosis infection: chronic productive cough, weight loss, night sweats, blood in sputum for >2 weeks	**	A17. Red flags of lower respiratory disease
Blood in the urine or sperm: refer all cases in men. Refer in women except in the case of acute urinary infection, in which case it is usually benign	**/*	A29. Red flags of diseases of the kidneys A30. Red flags of diseases of the ureters, bladder and urethra

TABLE B5 Red flags of disorders of the breast

Symptoms suggestive of:	Priority	For more detail and definitions go to:
Mastitis in pregnancy or puerperium: if not responding to treatment in 2 days or if features of an abscess (inflamed mass with severe malaise) present	**/*	A38. Red flags of the puerperium A39. Red flags of diseases of the breast
Inflamed breast tissue but not breastfeeding: it is rare to develop inflammation if not breastfeeding; may suggest underlying tumour	**/*	A39. Red flags of diseases of the breast
Insufficient breast milk: if the mother is considering stopping breastfeeding because of insufficient milk, refer to midwife for breastfeeding advice, as once a baby becomes reliant on formula milk it is often an irreversible decision	**/*	A38. Red flags of the puerperium
Lump in the breast: always refer for investigation. One in 10 breast lumps is cancerous	*	A39. Red flags of diseases of the breast
Eczema of nipple region: may be due to Bowen's disease (form of breast cancer)	*	A39. Red flags of diseases of the breast
Lactation but not breastfeeding: might suggest pituitary disorder	*	A39. Red flags of diseases of the breast
Hypopituitarism: inappropriate lactation, loss of libido, infertility, menstrual disturbances, tiredness, low blood pressure	*	A33. Red flags of other endocrine diseases

TABLE B6 Red flags of breathlessness or difficulty in breathing (see also B12: red flags of cough)

Symptoms suggestive of:	Priority	For more detail and definitions go to:
Severe asthma: at least two of the following – rapidly worsening breathlessness, >30 respirations/minute (or more if a child[1]), heart rate >110 beats/minute, reluctance to talk because of breathlessness, need to sit upright and still to assist breathing. Cyanosis is a very serious sign	***	A17. Red flags of lower respiratory disease
Infection of the alveoli (pneumonia): cough, fever, malaise, >30 respirations/minute (or more if a child[1]), heart rate >110 beats/minute, reluctance to talk because of breathlessness, need to sit upright and still to assist breathing. Cyanosis is a very serious sign	***/**	A17. Red flags of lower respiratory disease
Progression of respiratory infection to the lower respiratory tract: breathlessness with malaise suggests the involvement of the bronchi or lower air passages. Usually accompanied by cough and fever, but may be the only symptom of an infection in the elderly or immunocompromised	***/**	A16. Red flags of upper respiratory disease
Pulmonary embolism: sudden onset of pleurisy (chest pain exacerbated by breathing in), with breathlessness, cyanosis, collapse and blood in sputum	***	A17. Red flags of lower respiratory disease
Sudden lung collapse (pneumothorax): onset of severe breathlessness, may be some pleurisy (chest pain exacerbated by breathing in) and collapse if very severe	***	A17. Red flags of lower respiratory disease
Stridor (harsh noisy breathing heard on both the inbreath and outbreath): suggests obstruction to upper airway. Patient will want to sit upright and be still. Don't ask to examine the tongue	***/**	A16. Red flags of upper respiratory disease
Any new onset of difficulty breathing in a young child (<8 years old): possible asthma (suggested by the presence of cough), chest infection, foreign body in airway, allergic reaction. All need assessing, but some may require urgent treatment	***/**/*	A16. Red flags of upper respiratory disease
Unstable angina or heart attack: sustained intense chest pain associated with fear or dread. Palpitations and breathlessness may be present. The patient may vomit or develop a cold sweat. *Beware:* in the elderly can present as sudden onset of breathlessness, palpitations or confusion, but without pain	***	A13. Red flags of angina and heart attack

TABLE B6 Continued

Symptoms suggestive of:	Priority	For more detail and definitions go to:
Acute heart failure: sudden onset of disabling breathlessness and watery cough	***	A14. Red flags of heart failure and arrhythmias
Any sudden or gradual onset of muscle weakness that might be affecting muscles of respiration: needs to be referred urgently, as condition may progress to respiratory failure	***	A25. Red flags of diseases of the spinal cord and peripheral nerves
Severe chronic heart failure: marked swelling of ankles and lower legs, disabling breathlessness, cough and exhaustion. There may also be palpitations and chest pain on exertion	**	A14. Red flags of heart failure and arrhythmias
Mild chronic heart failure: slight swelling of ankles, slight breathlessness on exertion and when lying flat, cough, but no palpitations or chest pain	*	A14. Red flags of heart failure and arrhythmias
Stable angina: central chest pain related to exertion, eating or the cold which improves with rest. Pain is heavy and gripping (rather than sharp or stabbing), and can radiate down neck and arms *Beware:* in the elderly can present as episodes of breathlessness/chest tightness, but without pain	**/*	A13. Red flags of angina and heart attack
Complicated pericarditis: sharp central chest pain that is worse on leaning forward and lying down. Fever. Associated palpitations and breathlessness are more serious features	**	A15. Red flags of pericarditis
Pleurisy: localised chest pain which is associated with inspiration and expiration. Refer if associated with fever and breathlessness, as this is an indication of underlying pneumonia	**	A17. Red flags of lower respiratory disease
Long-standing anaemia: pallor, tiredness, breathlessness on exertion, feeling of faintness, depression, sore mouth and tongue	**/*	A18. Red flags of anaemia
Unexplained persistent blockage of nostril on one side: in an adult this suggests possible nasopharyngeal carcinoma; refer for investigations if persisting for >3 weeks In a child this suggests obstruction by a foreign body; refer as a high priority	*/**	A16. Red flags of upper respiratory disease A40. Red flags of childhood diseases

[1]Categorisation of respiratory rate in children:

The normal range for respiratory rate in children varies according to age.

The following rates indicate moderate to severe breathlessness:

newborn (0–3 months)	>60 breaths/minute
infant (3 months to 2 years)	>50 breaths/minute
young child (2–8 years)	>40 breaths/minute
older child to adult	>30 breaths/minute

TABLE B7 Red flags of bruising and purpura[1]

Symptoms suggestive of:	Priority	For more detail and definitions go to:
Bone marrow failure: severe progressive anaemia, recurrent progressive infections or bruising, purpura and bleeding	***/**	A1. Red flags of cancer A20. Red flags of leukaemia and lymphoma
Severe headache with fever and with a bruising and non-blanching rash: suggests meningococcal meningitis	***	A23. Red flags of headache
Bruising and non-blanching rash with severe malaise: suggests meningococcal septicaemia	***	A11. Red flags of diseases of the blood vessels
Purpura or bruising rash (non-blanching): suggests a bleeding disorder or vasculitis	***/**	A41. Red flags of diseases of the skin
Oedema, bruising and confusion in someone with known liver disease: suggests liver disease has progressed to a serious stage, and the patient is at risk of coma	**	A8. Red flags of diseases of the liver
Severe anaemia: extreme tiredness and breathlessness on exertion, excessive bruising and severe visual disturbances. There may also be features of strain on the cardiovascular system: chest pain on exertion, tachycardia and increasing oedema	**	A18. Red flags of anaemia

[1]Purpura is pinpoint bruising that appears as a rash of small, red, non-blanching macules. It may result from low platelets or from inflammation of the blood vessels (vasculitis).

TABLE B8 Red flags of chest pain

Symptoms suggestive of:	Priority	For more detail and definitions go to:
Unstable angina or heart attack: sustained intense chest pain associated with fear or dread. Palpitations and breathlessness may be present. The patient may vomit or develop a cold sweat *Beware:* in the elderly can present as sudden onset of breathlessness, palpitations or confusion, but without pain	***	A13. Red flags of angina and heart attack
Pulmonary embolism: sudden onset of pleurisy (chest pain related to breathing in) with breathlessness, cyanosis, collapse and blood in sputum	***	A17. Red flags of lower respiratory disease
Sudden lung collapse (pneumothorax): breathlessness; may be some pleurisy and collapse if very severe	***	A17. Red flags of lower respiratory disease

TABLE B8 Continued

Symptoms suggestive of:	Priority	For more detail and definitions go to:
Complicated pericarditis: sharp central chest pain that is worse on leaning forward and lying down. Fever. Associated palpitations and breathlessness are more serious features	***/**	A15. Red flags of pericarditis
Dissecting aortic aneurysm: sudden onset, tearing chest pain with radiation to back. Features of shock may be present (faintness, low blood pressure, rapid pulse)	***	A13. Red flags of angina and heart attack
Stable angina: central chest pain related to exertion, eating or the cold and which improves with rest. Pain is heavy and gripping (rather than sharp or stabbing), and can radiate down neck and arms *Beware:* in the elderly can present as episodes of breathlessness/chest tightness, but without pain	**/*	A13. Red flags of angina and heart attack
Uncomplicated pericarditis: sharp central chest pain which is worse on leaning forward and lying down. Fever should be slight and pulse rate no more than 100 beats/minute	**	A15. Red flags of pericarditis
Pleurisy: localised chest pain that is associated with inspiration and expiration. Refer if associated with breathlessness, as this is an indication of associated pneumonia or pulmonary embolism	**	A17. Red flags of lower respiratory disease
New onset of chronic cough or deep persistent chest pain in a smoker: this could be the first sign of **bronchial carcinoma**	**/*	A17. Red flags of lower respiratory disease
Early shingles: intense, one-sided pain, with overlying rash of crops of fluid-filled reddened and crusting blisters. The pain may precede the rash by 1–2 days. Refer for early consideration of antiviral treatment	**	A25. Red flags of diseases of the spinal cord and peripheral nerves

TABLE B9 Red flags particular to childhood diseases

This table lists only those red flags that are particular to children. Many of the red flags listed in the other tables also apply to children, and these are not repeated here.

Symptoms suggestive of:	Priority	For more detail and definitions go to:
Dehydration in an infant: dry mouth and skin, loss of skin turgor (firmness), drowsiness, sunken fontanelle (soft spot in region of Du24) and dry nappies	***/**	A40. Red flags of childhood diseases
Febrile convulsion in child: ongoing	***	A40. Red flags of childhood diseases

TABLE B9 Continued

Severe diarrhoea and vomiting if lasting >24 hours in infants	***/**	A6. Red flags of diseases of the stomach
High fever in a child (<8 years old) not responding to treatment within 2 hours	**	A40. Red flags of childhood diseases
Any fever if present in an infant (especially if <3 months old): treat with caution; may be the only sign of serious disease	**	A2. Red flags of infectious diseases: vulnerable groups
Febrile convulsion in child: recovered	**	A40. Red flags of childhood diseases
Complications of acute otitis media: persistent fever/pain/confusion for >3–4 days after the onset of the earache (may indicate spread of the infection, e.g. mastoiditis or brain abscess)	**	A40. Red flags of childhood diseases
Mastoiditis: fever, with a painful and swollen mastoid bone	**	A43. Red flags of diseases of the ear
Discharge from the eye: if severe, prolonged for >5 days and painful, or if seen in the newborn or a malnourished child	**	A42. Red flags of diseases of the eye
Malabsorption syndrome: loose, pale stools and malnutrition; weight loss, thin hair, dry skin, cracked lips and peeled tongue. Will present as failure to thrive in children	**/*	A7. Red flags of diseases of the pancreas A10. Red flags of diseases of the small and large intestines
Unexplained injury; child not thriving; child miserable: refer any situation in which you suspect the possibility of physical or sexual abuse as a high priority If in the UK, call the NSPCC helpline or the local Safeguarding Board for confidential advice in the first instance	**	A40. Red flags of childhood diseases
Vaginal discharge or itch before puberty: refer any situation in which you suspect the possibility of sexual abuse as a high priority If in the UK, call the NSPCC helpline or the local Safeguarding Board for confidential advice in the first instance	**	A40. Red flags of childhood diseases
Epilepsy: refer any child who has suffered a suspected blank episode (absence) or seizure	*	A40. Red flags of childhood diseases
New onset of difficulty hearing in a child: if lasting for >3 weeks (especially if interfering with school and social interactions)	*	A40. Red flags of childhood diseases
Squint: in any child if previously undiagnosed	*	A40. Red flags of childhood diseases
Soiling of stool (in underwear or bed): if affecting a previously continent child	*	A40. Red flags of childhood diseases
Bedwetting: if persisting over age 5 years	*	A40. Red flags of childhood diseases

TABLE B9 Continued

Symptoms suggestive of:	Priority	For more detail and definitions go to:
Primary amenorrhoea: no first menstrual period by 16th birthday	*	A34. Red flags of menstruation
Delayed puberty: secondary sexual characteristics not apparent by age 15 years in girls and 16 years in boys	*	A36. Red flags of structural disorders of the reproductive system
Precocious puberty: secondary sexual characteristics before age 8 years in girls and 9 years in boys	*	A36. Red flags of structural disorders of the reproductive system
Autism in a child: slow development of speech, impaired social interactions, little imaginative play, obsessional repetitive behaviour	*	A40. Red flags of childhood diseases

TABLE B10 Red flags of collapse and loss of consciousness (see also B11: red flags of confusion and clouding of consciousness)

Symptoms suggestive of:	Priority	More detail
Cardiac arrest: collapse with no palpable pulse	***	A14. Red flags of heart failure and arrhythmias
Loss of consciousness (continuing loss of neurological function): diverse causes include stroke, metabolic disease, brain infection, intoxication	***	A22. Red flags of brain haemorrhage, stroke and brain tumour
Rapid increase in intracranial pressure (intracranial haemorrhage): headache followed by a rapid deterioration of consciousness leading to coma. Irregular breathing patterns and pinpoint pupils are a very serious sign. May be spontaneous or may result from a head injury	***	A21. Red flags of raised intracranial pressure A22. Red flags of brain haemorrhage, stroke and brain tumour
First ever epileptic seizure: generalised tonic–clonic seizure: convulsions, loss of consciousness, bitten tongue, emptying of bladder and/or bowels. This is an emergency if the fit does not settle down within 2 minutes. Refer as high priority if fit has settled down	***	A24. Red flags of dementia, epilepsy and other disorders of the central nervous system
A severe headache that develops over the course of a few hours to days with fever, together with either vomiting or neck stiffness. The patient may become drowsy or unconscious. Suggests acute meningitis or encephalitis	***	A23 Red flags of headache
Febrile convulsion in child: ongoing	***	A3. Red flags of infectious diseases: fever, dehydration and confusion

TABLE B10 Continued

Symptoms suggestive of:	Priority	More detail
Confusion/coma with dehydration (hyperglycaemia)	***	A32. Red flags of diabetes mellitus
Hypoglycaemia (due to effects of insulin or antidiabetic medication in excess of bodily requirements): agitation, sweating, dilated pupils, confusion and coma	***	A32. Red flags of diabetes mellitus
Pulmonary embolism: sudden onset of pleurisy (chest pain on breathing in) with breathlessness, cyanosis, collapse	***	A17. Red flags of lower respiratory disease
Sudden lung collapse (pneumothorax): onset of severe breathlessness, may be some pleurisy (chest pain on breathing in) and collapse if very severe	***	A17. Red flags of lower respiratory disease
General symptoms of shock: dizziness, fainting and confusion. Rapid pulse of >100 beats/minute. Blood pressure <90/60 mmHg. Cold and clammy extremities. Refer if these symptoms are worsening or sustained (more than a few seconds)	***	A19. Red flags of haemorrhage and shock
Addison's disease: increased pigmentation of skin, weight loss, muscle wasting, tiredness, loss of libido, low blood pressure, diarrhoea and vomiting, confusion, collapse with dehydration	***/**	A33. Red flags of other endocrine diseases
Febrile convulsion in child: recovered	**	A40. Red flags of childhood diseases
Unexplained falls or faints in elderly person: may be the result of an arrhythmia **(cardiac syncope)**	**/*	A14 Red flags of heart failure and arrhythmias
A temporary loss of neurological function (usually <2 hours long): recovery from loss of consciousness, loss of vision, unsteadiness, confusion, loss of memory, loss of sensation or limb weakness	**	A22. Red flags of brain haemorrhage, stroke and brain tumour
Simple fainting: dizziness, temporary collapse (no more than a few seconds) and temporary confusion. Normal or slowed pulse rate. Blood pressure <90/60 mmHg. Cold and clammy extremities. Patient starts to recover in seconds to a minute. No need to refer	–	A19. Red flags of haemorrhage and shock

TABLE B11 Red flags of confusion and clouding of consciousness (see also B10: red flags of collapse and loss of consciousness)

Symptoms suggestive of:	Priority	For more detail and definitions go to:
General symptoms of shock: dizziness, fainting and confusion. Rapid pulse of >100 beats/minute. Blood pressure <90/60 mmHg. Cold and clammy extremities. Refer if these symptoms are worsening or sustained (more than a few seconds)	***	A19. Red flags of haemorrhage and shock
Hypoglycaemia (due to effects of insulin or antidiabetic medication in excess of bodily requirements): agitation, sweating, dilated pupils, confusion and coma	***	A32. Red flags of diabetes mellitus
Confusion/coma with dehydration (hyperglycaemia)	***	A32. Red flags of diabetes mellitus
Unusual drowsiness in infants (especially if <3 months old): may signify underlying serious illness	***/**	A2. Red flags of infectious diseases: vulnerable groups
Organic mental health disorder (a mental health condition due to an underlying gross physical cause): acute confusion, agitation, visual hallucinations, deterioration in intellectual skills, loss of ability to care for self. (These suggest organic brain disorder such as metabolic disease, drug intoxication, brain damage or dementia)	***/**	A44. Red flags of mental health disorders
A persisting loss of neurological function: including loss of vision, unsteadiness, confusion, loss of memory, loss of sensation or muscle weakness (possible stroke or multiple sclerosis)	***	A22. Red flags of brain haemorrhage, stroke and brain tumour A24. Red flags of dementia, epilepsy and other disorders of the central nervous system
Hallucinations, delusions or other evidence of thought disorder together with evidence of deteriorating self-care and personality change: all are features of a psychosis such as schizophrenia. Suicide risk is high	***/**	A44. Red flags of mental health disorders
Mania: increasing agitation, grandiosity, pressure of speech and sleeplessness with delusional thinking: all are features of bipolar disorder, a form of psychosis that carries a high risk of behaviour that can be both socially and physically damaging to the patient. Suicide risk is high	***/**	A44. Red flags of mental health disorders
Post-natal psychosis: delusional or paranoid ideas and hallucinations are key features. This condition is associated with a high risk of suicide or harm to the baby	***/**	A38. Red flags of the puerperium

TABLE B11 Continued

Symptoms suggestive of:	Priority	For more detail and definitions go to:
Acute confusion in an elderly person: can result from an underlying medical condition, such as stroke, heart attack, infection or pain	***/**	A2. Red flags of infectious diseases: vulnerable groups
Confusion in older children and adults with fever	**	A3. Red flags of infectious diseases: fever, dehydration and confusion
Slow increase in intracranial pressure: progressive headaches and vomiting over the timescale of a few weeks to months. The headaches are worse in the morning and the vomiting may be effortless. Blurring of vision and confusion may be additional symptoms	**	A21. Red flags of raised intracranial pressure
Loss of neurological function which is progressive over the course of days to weeks: may include confusion. This is more suggestive of a brain tumour than a stroke	**	A22. Red flags of brain haemorrhage, stroke and brain tumour
Pernicious anaemia: tiredness, lemon-yellow pallor and gradual onset of neurological symptoms (numbness, weakness, confusion)	**/*	A18. Red flags of anaemia
A temporary loss of neurological function (usually <2 hours long): recovery from loss of consciousness, loss of vision, unsteadiness, confusion, loss of memory, loss of sensation or limb weakness (possible transient ischaemic attack (TIA))	**/*	A22. Red flags of brain haemorrhage, stroke and brain tumour A24. Red flags of dementia, epilepsy and other disorders of the central nervous system
Progressive decline in mental and social functioning: increasing difficulty in intellectual function, memory, concentration and use of language	*	A22. Red flags of brain haemorrhage, stroke and brain tumour A24. Red flags of dementia, epilepsy and other disorders of the central nervous system
First ever epileptic seizure (complex partial): generalised absence or complex partial seizures: defined periods of vagueness or loss of awareness, or mood or personality changes. Refer any child who has suffered a suspected blank episode (absence) or seizure	*	A24. Red flags of dementia, epilepsy and other disorders of the central nervous system
Simple fainting: dizziness, temporary collapse (no more than a few seconds) and temporary confusion. Normal or slowed pulse rate. Blood pressure <90/60 mmHg. Cold and clammy extremities. Patient starts to recover in seconds to a minute. No need to refer	–	A19. Red flags of haemorrhage and shock

TABLE B12 Red flags of cough (see also B6: red flags of breathlessness and difficulty breathing)

Symptoms suggestive of:	Priority	For more detail and definitions go to:
Acute heart failure: sudden onset of disabling breathlessness and watery cough	***	A14. Red flags of heart failure and arrhythmias
Infection of the alveoli (pneumonia): cough, fever, malaise, >30 respirations/minute (or more if a child[1]), heart rate >110 beats/minute, reluctance to talk because of breathlessness, need to sit upright and be still to assist breathing. Cyanosis is a very serious sign	***/**	A17. Red flags of lower respiratory disease
Progression of infection to the lower respiratory tract: breathlessness[1] with malaise suggests the involvement of the bronchi or lower air passages. Usually accompanied by cough and fever, but may be the only symptom of an infection in the elderly or immunocompromised	***/**	A16. Red flags of upper respiratory disease
Any new onset of difficulty breathing in a young child (<8 years old): possible asthma (suggested by coughing as well as difficulty breathing), chest infection, foreign body in airway, allergic reaction. All need assessing, but some may require urgent treatment	***/**/*	A16. Red flags of upper respiratory disease
Progressive upper respiratory infection in susceptible people (e.g. the frail elderly, the immunocompromised and people with pre-existing disease of the bronchi and bronchioles): cough and fever, or new production of yellow–green phlegm, each persisting for >3 days	**	A16. Red flags of upper respiratory disease A17. Red flags of lower respiratory disease
Tuberculosis infection: chronic productive cough, weight loss, night sweats, blood in sputum for >2 weeks	**	A17. Red flags of lower respiratory disease
New onset of chronic cough or deep persistent chest pain in a smoker	**/*	A17. Red flags of lower respiratory disease
Severe chronic heart failure: marked swelling of ankles and lower legs, disabling breathlessness, cough and exhaustion. There may also be palpitations and chest pain on exertion	**	A14. Red flags of heart failure and arrhythmias
Coughing up of blood (haemoptysis): (if on only a single occasion, only amounts more than a teaspoon in volume are significant)	**	A17. Red flags of lower respiratory disease

TABLE B12 Continued

Symptoms suggestive of:	Priority	For more detail and definitions go to:
Mild chronic heart failure: slight swelling of ankles, slight breathlessness on exertion and when lying flat, cough, but no palpitations or chest pain. Dry cough may be the only symptom in sedentary elderly people	*	A14. Red flags of heart failure and arrhythmias

[1]Categorisation of respiratory rate in adults:
– Normal respiratory rate in an adult: 10–20 breaths/minute (one breath is one inhalation and exhalation).
– Moderate breathlessness in an adult: >30 breaths/minute.
– Severe breathlessness in an adult: >60 breaths/minute.

Categorisation of respiratory rate in children:

The normal range for respiratory rate in children varies according to age.

The following rates indicate moderate to severe breathlessness:

newborn (0–3 months)	>60 breaths/minute
infant (3 months to 2 years)	>50 breaths/minute
young child (2–8 years)	>40 breaths/minute
older child to adult	>30 breaths/minute

TABLE B13 Red flags of dehydration

Symptoms suggestive of:	Priority	For more detail and definitions go to:
Dehydration in an infant: signs include dry mouth and skin, loss of skin turgor (firmness), drowsiness, sunken fontanelle (soft spot in the region of acupoint Du24) and dry nappies	***/**	A3. Red flags of infectious diseases: fever, dehydration and confusion
Type 1 diabetes or poorly controlled type 2 diabetes: short history of thirst, weight loss and excessive urination, which is rapidly progressive in severity. Can progress to confusion/coma, with dehydration (due to hyperglycaemia)	***/**	A32. Red flags of diabetes mellitus
Addison's disease: increased pigmentation of skin, weight loss, muscle wasting, tiredness, loss of libido, low blood pressure, diarrhoea and vomiting, confusion, collapse with dehydration	***/**	A33. Red flags of other endocrine diseases
Dehydration in older children and adults if severe or lasting >48 hours: signs include dry mouth and skin, loss of skin turgor, low blood pressure, dizziness on standing and poor urine output	**	A3. Red flags of infectious diseases: fever, dehydration and confusion

TABLE B14 Red flags of depression and exhaustion

Symptoms suggestive of:	Priority	For more detail and definitions go to:
Suicidal thoughts with features that suggest serious risk: old age, male sex, social isolation, concrete plans in place	**	A44. Red flags of mental health disorders
Severe anaemia: extreme tiredness and breathlessness on exertion, excessive bruising and severe visual disturbances. There may also be features of strain on the cardiovascular system: chest pain on exertion, features of tachycardia and increasing oedema	**	A18. Red flags of anaemia
Long-standing anaemia: pallor, tiredness, breathlessness on exertion, feeling of faintness, depression, sore mouth and tongue	**/*	A18. Red flags of anaemia
Type 2 diabetes: general feeling of unwellness, with thirst and increased need to urinate large amounts of urine, which develop over the course of weeks to months	**/*	A32. Red flags of diabetes mellitus
Pernicious anaemia: tiredness, lemon-yellow pallor and gradual onset of neurological symptoms (numbness, weakness, confusion)	**/*	A18. Red flags of anaemia
Hypopituitarism: loss of libido, infertility, menstrual disturbances, tiredness, low blood pressure, inappropriate lactation	**/*	A33. Red flags of other endocrine diseases
Postnatal depression lasting >3 weeks which is not responding to your treatment: refer straight away if the woman is experiencing suicidal ideas, or if you believe the health of the baby to be at risk	**	A38. Red flags of the puerperium
Hypothyroidism (symptoms and signs tend to be progressive over the course of a few months). Symptoms: tiredness, depression, weight gain, heavy periods, constipation and cold intolerance. Signs: dry puffy skin, dry and thin hair, slow pulse	*	A31. Red flags of diseases of the thyroid gland
Severe disturbance of body image: if not responding to your treatment, and resulting in features of progressive anorexia nervosa or bulimia nervosa (progressive weight loss, secondary amenorrhoea, or repeated compulsion to bring about vomiting)	*	A44. Red flags of mental health disorders

TABLE B15 Red flags of dizziness

Dizziness is used often by patients to mean lightheadedness. True 'vertigo' is the medical term used to describe a sensation of dizziness in which the world appears to be spinning. The patient may lose balance or feel acutely nauseous. The term 'vertigo' is also sometimes used to mean fear of heights; but strictly speaking should only be used to describe a state in which there is a sensation of movement.
It is important diagnostically to distinguish dizziness from true vertigo.

Symptoms suggestive of:	Priority	For more detail and definitions go to:
Shock: dizziness, fainting and confusion. Rapid pulse of >100 beats/minute. Blood pressure <90/60 mmHg. Cold and clammy extremities. Refer if these symptoms are worsening or sustained (more than a few seconds)	***	A19. Red flags of haemorrhage and shock
Vertigo in young person: usually due to benign labyrinthitis and will settle down. Refer if lasting >6 weeks or if so severe as to be causing recurrent vomiting. Refer if patient is at increased risk of thromboembolic disease (e.g. in pregnancy) so that the possibility of stroke can be excluded	**/*	A43. Red flags of diseases of the ear
Vertigo for the first time in older person (>45 years old): refer for high priority medical opinion. Stroke is a more likely cause in this age group. If the vertigo is persisting and profound, refer urgently	**/***	A43. Red flags of diseases of the ear
Simple fainting: dizziness, temporary collapse (no more than a few seconds) and temporary confusion. Normal or slowed pulse rate. Blood pressure <90/60 mmHg. Cold and clammy extremities. Patient starts to recover in seconds to a minute. No need to refer	–	A19. Red flags of haemorrhage and shock

TABLE B16 Red flags of diseases of the ear

Symptoms suggestive of:	Priority	For more detail and definitions go to:
Sudden onset of absolute deafness (one-sided or bilateral): needs same-day, specialist assessment	**	A43. Red flags of diseases of the ear
Complications of acute otitis media: persistent fever/pain/confusion for >3–4 days after the onset of the earache (may indicate spread of the infection, e.g. mastoiditis or brain abscess)	**	A43. Red flags of diseases of the ear
Mastoiditis: fever, with a painful and swollen mastoid bone. Serious infection; needs same-day assessment and treatment	**	A43. Red flags of diseases of the ear
Earache in an adult for >3 weeks: may suggest nasopharyngeal pathology; refer to exclude cancer	*	A43. Red flags of diseases of the ear

TABLE B16 Continued

Symptoms suggestive of:	Priority	For more detail and definitions go to:
Persistent discharge (lasting >2 weeks) from the ear (chronic otitis media/otitis externa): risk of permanent damage to ear from chronic inflammation; refer for assessment and treatment	*	A43. Red flags of diseases of the ear
Gradual onset of relative deafness in adult for >7 days (exclude earwax as a cause if possible): deafness from respiratory infection should have cleared by this time; refer to exclude progressive cause, including acoustic neuroma	*	A43. Red flags of diseases of the ear
Tinnitus, if progressive (constant or variable tinnitus is common and usually benign): refer to exclude progressive cause, including acoustic neuroma	*	A43. Red flags of diseases of the ear
New onset of difficulty hearing in a child lasting for >3 weeks (especially if interfering with school and social interactions): prolonged deafness can affect the development of a child; refer for assessment and treatment if not responding to yours	*	A43. Red flags of diseases of the ear

TABLE B17 Red flags of diseases of the eye

Symptoms suggestive of:	Priority	For more detail and definitions go to:
Painful, red and swollen eyes and eyelids: patient (often a child) very unwell (orbital cellulitis)	***	A42. Red flags of diseases of the eye
Sudden onset of painless blurring or loss of sight in one or both eyes accompanied by one-sided headache in patient >50 years old: suggestive of temporal arteritis; high risk of further loss of sight or stroke. Refer for urgent treatment with corticosteroids	***	A42. Red flags of diseases of the eye
An intensely painful and red eye: iritis, choroiditis, acute glaucoma, corneal ulcer or keratitis	***/**	A42. Red flags of diseases of the eye
Sudden onset of painless blurring or loss of sight in one or both eyes: refer as soon as possible, as may result from treatable retinal tear	***/**	A42. Red flags of diseases of the eye
A painful eye with no obvious inflammation: deep, intense pain exacerbated by eye movement is characteristic of optic neuritis or choroiditis	**	A42. Red flags of diseases of the eye
Foreign body in the eye	**	A42. Red flags of diseases of the eye
Inability to close the eye: occurs in severe Bell's palsy or thyroid eye disease. The conjunctiva is at risk of ulceration	**	A42. Red flags of diseases of the eye
Recent onset of double vision in an adult	**	A42. Red flags of diseases of the eye

TABLE B17 Continued

Symptoms suggestive of:	Priority	For more detail and definitions go to:
Discharge from the eye: if severe, prolonged for >5 days and painful, or if seen in the following vulnerable groups: • the newborn • the immunocompromised • malnourished people	**	A42. Red flags of diseases of the eye
Gradual onset of painless blurring or loss of sight in one or both eyes: possible refractive error, cataract, glaucoma or macular degeneration	*	A42. Red flags of diseases of the eye
Thyroid eye disease: staring eyes (whites visible above and below pupils), inflamed conjunctivae, symptoms of hyperthyroidism (tremor, agitation, weight loss, palpitations)	*	A42. Red flags of diseases of the eye
Squint: in any child if previously undiagnosed	*	A42. Red flags of diseases of the eye
Recent onset of drooping eyelid (ptosis)	*	A42. Red flags of diseases of the eye

TABLE B18 Red flags of fever

Symptoms suggestive of:	Priority	For more detail and definitions go to:
Meningococcal septicaemia: acute onset of a purpuric rash, possibly accompanied by headache, vomiting and fever	***	A11. Red flags of diseases of the blood vessels
A severe headache that develops over the course of a few hours to days, with fever, and together with either vomiting or neck stiffness: suggests acute meningitis or encephalitis	***	A23. Red flags of headache
Febrile convulsion in child: ongoing	***	A3. Red flags of infectious diseases: fever, dehydration and confusion
Fever of any level in an immunocompromised person: treat with caution, as could be the only sign of serious infection. Refer if you have any uncertainty about the case	**	A2. Red flags of infectious diseases: vulnerable groups
High fever in a child (<8 years old) if high (>38.5°C) and not responding to treatment within 2 hours	**	A3. Red flags of infectious diseases: fever, dehydration and confusion
Fever in pregnancy if high (>38.5°C) and no response to treatment in 24 hours: refer early, as risk to fetus	**	A37. Red flags of pregnancy

TABLE B18 Continued

Symptoms suggestive of:	Priority	For more detail and definitions go to:
Fever in the puerperium: any case of fever developing in the first 2 weeks of the puerperium (temperature >38°C for >24 hours). Refer early, as possible uterine infection	**	A38. Red flags of the puerperium
Fever of any level in an infant (especially if <3 months old): treat with caution, as could be the only sign of serious underlying disease. Refer if you have any uncertainty about the case	**	A2. Red flags of infectious diseases: vulnerable groups
Fever of any level in an elderly person: treat with caution, as could be the only sign of serious underlying disease. Refer if you have any uncertainty about the case	**	A2. Red flags of infectious diseases: vulnerable groups
Fever of any level in anyone with a recent history of travel to a tropical country (within the past month): treat with caution, as could be a sign of tropical disease. Refer if you have any uncertainty about the case	**	A2. Red flags of infectious diseases: vulnerable groups
High fever in an older child or adult (>38.5°C) which does not respond to treatment within 48 hours	**	A3. Red flags of infectious diseases: fever, dehydration and confusion
Any fever that persists or recurs over >2 weeks: possible chronic infection, inflammatory process or cancer	**	A1. Red flags of cancer A3. Red flags of infectious diseases: fever, dehydration and confusion
Febrile convulsion in child: recovered	**	A3. Red flags of infectious diseases: fever, dehydration and confusion

TABLE B19 Red flags of headache

Symptoms suggestive of:	Priority	For more detail and definitions go to:
A sudden very severe headache that comes on out of the blue: the patient needs to lie down, and may vomit. There may be neck stiffness (reluctance to move the head) and dislike of bright light. This suggests subarachnoid (intracranial) haemorrhage	***	A23. Red flags of headache
Severe headache that develops over the course of a few hours to days with fever, together with either vomiting or neck stiffness: there may be a bruising and non-blanching rash. Suggests acute meningitis or encephalitis	***	A23. Red flags of headache
Malignant hypertension: diastolic hypertension >120 mmHg, with symptoms including recently worsening headaches, blurred vision, chest pain	***/**	A12. Red flags of hypertension

TABLE B19 Continued

Symptoms suggestive of:	Priority	For more detail and definitions go to:
Pre-eclampsia/HELLP syndromes: headache, abdominal pain, visual disturbance, nausea and vomiting and oedema (in middle to late pregnancy)	***	A37. Red flags of pregnancy
Severe, one-sided headache over the temple occurring for the first time in an elderly person or in someone with polymyalgia rheumatica: possible temporal arteritis. Blurring or loss of sight are very serious signs	***/**	A23. Red flags of headache
Long history of worsening (progressive) headaches: especially with generalised symptoms such as fever, loss of appetite, exhaustion or neurological symptoms. Suggests malignancy or brain abscess	**/*	A23. Red flags of headache
Slow increase in intracranial pressure: progressive headaches and vomiting over the timescale of a few weeks to months. The headaches are worse in the morning and the vomiting may be effortless. Blurring of vision and confusion may be additional symptoms	**	A21. Red flags of raised intracranial pressure A22. Red flags of brain haemorrhage, stroke and brain tumour
Growth of a pituitary tumour: progressive headaches, visual disturbance and double vision	**/*	A33. Red flags of other endocrine diseases
Acromegaly (growth hormone excess): thickening of facial features and soft tissues, enlarged hands and feet, headaches, high blood pressure	**/*	A33. Red flags of other endocrine diseases
Trigeminal neuralgia (and other forms of one-sided facial pain): lancinating pain, on one side of the face, which radiates out from a focal point in response to defined triggers. May be associated with twitching (tic douloureux)	*	A25. Red flags of diseases of the spinal cord and peripheral nerves

TABLE B20 Red flags of hypertension

Symptoms suggestive of:	Priority	For more detail and definitions go to:
Malignant hypertension: diastolic hypertension >120 mmHg, with symptoms including recently worsening headaches, blurred vision, chest pain	***/**	A12. Red flags of hypertension
Pre-eclampsia/HELLP syndromes: headache, abdominal pain, visual disturbance, nausea and vomiting, and oedema (in middle to late pregnancy). Often follows a rise in blood pressure	***	A34. Red flags of pregnancy
Seriously high hypertension: systolic pressure ≥220 mmHg, diastolic pressure ≥120 mmHg, but no symptoms	**	A12. Red flags of hypertension

TABLE B20 Continued

Symptoms suggestive of:	Priority	For more detail and definitions go to:
Moderate to severe pregnancy-induced hypertension: diastolic pressure >100 mmHg or systolic pressure >140 mmHg. Arrange same-day assessment with midwife	**	A37. Red flags of pregnancy
Severe hypertension: systolic pressure ≥180 mmHg, diastolic pressure ≥110 mmHg. Refer as high priority if major risk factors[1] are present. Otherwise, refer for treatment if there is no improvement in 2 weeks	*	A12. Red flags of hypertension
Moderate hypertension: systolic pressure ≥160 mmHg and <180 mmHg, diastolic pressure ≥100 mmHg and <110 mmHg. Refer for assessment if risk factors[1] are present, otherwise only refer if there is no improvement within 4 weeks	*	A12. Red flags of hypertension
Mild hypertension: systolic pressure ≥140 mmHg and <160 mmHg, diastolic pressure ≥90 mmHg and <100 mmHg. Refer for assessment if risk factors[1] are present, otherwise refer only if there is no improvement within 3 months	*	A12. Red flags of hypertension
Mild pregnancy-induced hypertension: diastolic pressure 90–99 mmHg, systolic pressure <140 mmHg	*	A37. Red flags of pregnancy
Potential pregnancy-induced hypertension: systolic pressure is 30 mmHg or diastolic pressure is 15 mmHg above any measurement taken previously in pregnancy	*	A37. Red flags of pregnancy
Hypertension of any level with established kidney disease	*	A12. Red flags of hypertension
Hypertension of any level with diabetes	*	A12. Red flags of hypertension
Cushing's syndrome: weight gain, weakness and wasting of limb muscles, stretch marks and bruises. Mood changes, hypertension, red cheeks, acne	*	A28. Red flags of other endocrine diseases
Acromegaly (growth hormone excess): thickening of facial features and soft tissues, enlarged hands and feet, headaches, high blood pressure	*	A28. Red flags of other endocrine diseases

[1]In this case, major risk factors are features that are known to be associated with increased risk of a cardiovascular event in the presence of hypertension. These include diabetes, past history of heart disease, chronic leg ischaemia and kidney disease.

TABLE B21 Red flags of infections

Symptoms suggestive of:	Priority	For more detail and definitions go to:
Bone marrow failure and current infection: severe progressive anaemia, recurrent progressive infections or bruising, purpura and bleeding	***/**	A1. Red flags of cancer A20. Red flags of leukaemia and lymphoma
Severe headache that develops over the course of a few hours to days with fever, together with either vomiting or neck stiffness: there may be a bruising and non-blanching rash. Suggests acute meningitis or encephalitis	***	A23. Red flags of headache
Pelvic inflammatory disease (acute form): low abdominal pain with collapse, fever	***	A35. Red flags of sexually transmitted diseases
Unexplained infection or spreading areas of inflammation in an infant (especially if <3 months old): treat with caution as the immune system is immature and infections can take hold easily	**	A2. Red flags of infectious diseases: vulnerable groups
Unexplained infection or spreading areas of inflammation in the elderly: treat with caution as the immune system is deficient and infections can take hold easily	**	A2. Red flags of infectious diseases: vulnerable groups
Unexplained infection or spreading areas of inflammation in an immunocompromised person: treat with caution as the immune system is deficient and infections can take hold easily	**	A2. Red flags of infectious diseases: vulnerable groups
Unexplained infections in pregnancy: treat with caution as certain infections can damage the embryo/fetus	**	A2. Red flags of infectious diseases: vulnerable groups
A rapidly advancing region or line of redness tracking up the skin of a limb (following the pathway of a lymphatic vessel): cellulitis and/or lymphangitis. Deep tissue infection; may need antibiotic treatment to prevent spread	**	A41. Red flags of diseases of the skin
A rapidly enlarging patch(es) of painful, crusting or swollen red skin: most likely to be a bacterial infection (impetigo or erysipelas). Very contagious, and may require antibiotic treatment if not settling down Refer with some urgency if this occurs in someone with eczema; possible viral infection causing the serious condition of eczema herpeticum	**	A41. Red flags of diseases of the skin
Generalised macular rash (flat red spots): refer if you suspect rubella, measles or scarlet fever (notifiable diseases)	**	A41. Red flags of diseases of the skin
Early shingles: intense, one-sided pain, with overlying rash of crops of fluid-filled reddened and crusting blisters. The pain may precede the rash by 1–2 days. Early antiviral therapy can reduce the severity of post-herpetic neuralgia; important to consider for elderly people	**	A41. Red flags of diseases of the skin

TABLE B21 Continued

Symptoms suggestive of:	Priority	For more detail and definitions go to:
Complications of acute otitis media: persistent fever/pain/confusion for >3–4 days after the onset of the earache (may indicate spread of the infection, e.g. mastoiditis or brain abscess)	**	A43. Red flags of diseases of the ear
Mastoiditis: fever, with a painful and swollen mastoid bone. This deep bone infection is unlikely to settle without antibiotic therapy	**	A43. Red flags of diseases of the ear
Discharge from the eye: if severe, prolonged for >5 days and painful, or if seen in the following vulnerable groups: • the newborn • the immunocompromised • malnourished people	**	A42. Red flags of diseases of the eye
Fever with rash in the first trimester of pregnancy: refer suspected rubella or chickenpox so that the health of the embryo/fetus can be monitored	**	A37. Red flags of pregnancy
Offensive, fishy, watery discharge in pregnancy (possible bacterial vaginosis): can increase risk of early labour	**	A35. Red flags of sexually transmitted diseases
Pelvic inflammatory disease (chronic form): vaginal discharge, gripy abdominal pain, pain on intercourse, dysmenorrhoea, infertility	**/*	A35. Red flags of sexually transmitted diseases
Fever with rash in the last trimester of pregnancy: refer if chickenpox or shingles suspected, as there is a risk of fatal fetal varicella infection	**	A37. Red flags of pregnancy
Discharge from penis: may indicate sexually transmitted disease	**	A35. Red flags of sexually transmitted diseases
Pronounced features of candidal infection (thrush) of the skin or mucous membranes of the mouth: suggests underlying diabetes or immune deficiency	*	A4. Red flags of diseases of the mouth A41. Red flags of diseases of the skin
Outbreak of genital herpes in the last trimester of pregnancy: refer as, if apparent during labour, herpes virus can be transmitted to the baby. Planned Caesarean section may be indicated	*	A35. Red flags of sexually transmitted diseases
Poor wound healing, especially in the feet and legs: might suggest diabetes mellitus or immune deficiency	**/*	A32. Red flags of diabetes mellitus
Increased tendency to infections such as cystitis, boils and oral thrush (candidiasis): might suggest diabetes mellitus or immune deficiency	*	A32. Red flags of diabetes mellitus

TABLE B22 Red flags of jaundice

Symptoms suggestive of:	Priority	For more detail and definitions go to:
Right hypochondriac pain that is very intense and comes in waves; associated with jaundice. Acute cholecystitis: may be associated with fever and vomiting. This is one of the manifestations of the acute abdomen	***/**	A9. Red flags of diseases of the gallbladder
Jaundice (yellowish skin, yellow whites of the eyes, and possibly dark urine and pale stools): itch may be a prominent symptom. Always refer any case of jaundice, as it more often than not results from serious disease of the liver, gallbladder, pancreas or blood	**	A7. Red flags of diseases of the pancreas A8. Red flags of diseases of the liver A9. Red flags of diseases of the gallbladder

TABLE B23 Red flags of lumps, masses and glands

Symptoms suggestive of:	Priority	For more detail and definitions go to:
A single, grossly enlarged tonsil: patient unwell, feverish and has foul-smelling breath. This suggests quinsy, which is a surgical emergency as breathing may be compromised	***/**	A16. Red flags of upper respiratory disease
Tender or inflamed gums or salivary glands which do not respond within days to your treatment	**	A4. Red flags of diseases of the mouth
Any unexplained lump >1 cm in diameter: especially if hard, irregular, fixed and painless	*	A1. Red flags of cancer
A single markedly enlarged lymph node (>2 cm in diameter) with no obvious cause and persisting for more than 2 weeks	*	A1. Red flags of cancer A20. Red flags of leukaemia and lymphoma
Multiple enlarged painless lymph nodes (>1 cm in diameter) with no other obvious cause (e.g. known glandular fever infection) and persisting for more than 2 weeks	*	A1. Red flags of cancer A20. Red flags of leukaemia and lymphoma
A single, grossly enlarged tonsil: patient generally well. If patient appears well, lymphoma is a possible diagnosis. Systemic symptoms may include fever, night sweats and weight loss	*	A16. Red flags of upper respiratory disease
Painless enlargement of a salivary gland over weeks to months: possible salivary tumour	*	A4. Red flags of diseases of the mouth
Painful or painless enlargement of a salivary gland immediately after eating: suggests salivary gland stone; refer if does not settle down in a week, or sooner if painful	*	A4. Red flags of diseases of the mouth

TABLE B23 Continued

Symptoms suggestive of:	Priority	For more detail and definitions go to:
Goitre: refer only if symptoms of hyperthyroidism or hypothyroidism are present, or if the goitre is tender, irregular or noticeably enlarging. Small, smooth, rubbery goitres are common and benign	*	A31. Red flags of diseases of the thyroid gland
Any lump in the breast: refer, as 1 in 10 of all breast lumps show malignant change	*	A39. Red flags of diseases of the breast
Any lump in the testis: refer as, although usually benign, early diagnosis of testicular cancer has a very good prognosis	*	A36. Red flags of structural disorders of the reproductive system
Breast tissue development in adult men (gynaecomastia): although common, benign and transitory in teenage boys, breast lumps in men should be referred to exclude cancer	*	A39. Red flags of diseases of the breast
Abdominal swelling: discrete mass in suprapubic or iliac fossa regions: possible fibroids, ovarian cyst, tumour, pregnancy	*	A36. Red flags of structural disorders of the reproductive system
Signs of an inguinal hernia: swelling in groin that is more pronounced on standing, especially if uncomfortable	*	A10. Red flags of disorders of the small and large intestines
Painless lump felt in anus: refer to exclude serious conditions of anal warts and anal carcinoma	*	A10. Red flags of disorders of the small and large intestines
Painful lump felt in anus: refer to exclude strangulated haemorrhoid, which will require a surgical opinion	**/*	A10. Red flags of disorders of the small and large intestines
Any lumps/moles with features suggestive of malignancy: recent change in size, irregularity of shape or pigmentation, a tendency to bleed, crusting, >5 mm in diameter, intense black colour	*	A41. Red flags of diseases of the skin

TABLE B24 Red flags of disorders of menstruation

Symptoms suggestive of:	Priority	For more detail and definitions go to:
Postpartum haemorrhage: refer if bleeding is any more than a blood-stained discharge after childbirth. A profuse bleed of >500 mL or the symptoms of shock (low blood pressure, fainting, rapid pulse rate) constitutes an emergency	***/**	A38. Red flags of the puerperium
Menorrhagia (heavy periods) with features of severe anaemia (tiredness, breathlessness, palpitations on exertion)	**	A34. Red flags of menstruation
Vaginal discharge: if irregular, blood-stained or unusual smell	**/*	A35. Red flags of sexually transmitted diseases

TABLE B24 Continued

Symptoms suggestive of:	Priority	For more detail and definitions go to:
Hyperthyroidism. Symptoms: irritability, anxiety, sleeplessness, increased appetite, loose stools, weight loss, scanty periods and heat intolerance. Signs: sweaty skin, tremor of the hands, staring eyes and rapid pulse	**/*	A31. Red flags of diseases of the thyroid gland
Post-menopausal bleeding: any unexplained bleeding after the menopause	*	A34. Red flags of menstruation
Pelvic inflammatory disease (chronic form): vaginal discharge, gripy abdominal pain, pain on intercourse, dysmenorrhoea (painful periods), infertility	*	A35. Red flags of sexually transmitted diseases
Primary amenorrhoea: after age 16 years No menstrual period by the time of the 16th birthday	*	A34. Red flags of menstruation
Secondary amenorrhoea: for >12 months Cessation of menstrual periods	*	A34. Red flags of menstruation
Metrorrhagia: bleeding between periods that has no regular pattern. This includes post-coital bleeding (bleeding after intercourse)	*	A34. Red flags of menstruation
Severe disturbance of body image: with features of progressive anorexia nervosa or bulimia nervosa (e.g. progressive weight loss, secondary amenorrhoea or repeated compulsion to bring about vomiting) and not responding to your treatment in 3 weeks	*	A44. Red flags of mental health disorders
Hypopituitarism: loss of libido, infertility, menstrual disturbances, tiredness, low blood pressure, inappropriate lactation	*	A33. Red flags of other endocrine diseases

TABLE B25 Red flags of disorders of the mouth

Symptoms suggestive of:	Priority	For more detail and definitions go to:
Painful ulceration of mouth: if persistent or if preventing proper hydration	**/*	A4. Red flags of diseases of the mouth
Enlarged or inflamed gums or salivary glands which do not respond within days to your treatment	**/*	A4. Red flags of diseases of the mouth
Long-standing anaemia: pallor, tiredness, breathlessness on exertion, feeling of faintness, depression, sore mouth and tongue	**/*	A18. Red flags of anaemia
Persistent oral thrush (candidiasis) (appearing as a thick white coating on tongue or palate): suggests underlying diabetes mellitus or immune deficiency	*	A4. Red flags of diseases of the mouth
Persistent, painless, white plaque (leukoplakia) on the tongue (appearing as a coat that appears to sit on the surface of the sides of the tongue): this is a pre-malignant change	*	A4. Red flags of diseases of the mouth

TABLE B26 Red flags of muscle tremor and spasms

Symptoms suggestive of:	Priority	For more detail and definitions go to:
Tremor with features of hyperthyroidism (symptoms and signs tend to be progressive over the course of a few months). Symptoms: irritability, anxiety, sleeplessness, increased appetite, loose stools, weight loss, scanty periods and heat intolerance. Signs: sweaty skin, staring eyes and rapid pulse	**/*	A31. Red flags of diseases of the thyroid gland
First ever epileptic seizure – focal simple seizures: episodes of coarse twitching of one part of the body	**	A22. Red flags of brain haemorrhage, stroke and brain tumour
Progressive coarse tremor appearing in middle to late life: possible Parkinson's or Huntingdon's disease (coarse tremor); distinguish from benign essential tremor (a fine tremor that worsens with anxiety), which does not require referral	*	A24. Red flags of dementia, epilepsy and other disorders of the central nervous system

TABLE B27 Red flags of numbness

Symptoms suggestive of:	Priority	For more detail and definitions go to:
An unexplained temporary loss of neurological function (usually <2 hours long): including loss of consciousness, loss of vision, unsteadiness, confusion, loss of memory, loss of sensation or limb weakness. This is a transient ischaemic attack (TIA) until proved otherwise. Could also be the first presentation of migrainous aura	**	A22. Red flags of brain haemorrhage, stroke and brain tumour A24. Red flags of dementia, epilepsy and other disorders of the central nervous system
A persisting loss of neurological function: including loss of vision, unsteadiness, confusion, loss of memory, loss of sensation or muscle weakness. This could be the result of a stroke, or a relapse of multiple sclerosis	**	A22. Red flags of brain haemorrhage, stroke and brain tumour A24. Red flags of dementia, epilepsy and other disorders of the central nervous system
A loss of neurological function that is progressive over the course of days to weeks: this is more suggestive of a brain tumour than a stroke	**	A22. Red flags of brain haemorrhage, stroke and brain tumour

TABLE B27 Continued

Symptoms suggestive of:	Priority	For more detail and definitions go to:
Any other sudden or gradual onset of unexplained severe numbness or pins and needles: all possible causes of polyneuropathy or mononeuropathy merit investigation. However, if symptoms suggest benign nerve root impingement (i.e. numbness affecting hand or arm or back of leg down to foot of one side only in association with neck or low back pain or muscle spasm) then no need to refer straight away	**	A25. Red flags of diseases of the spinal cord and peripheral nerves
Intervertebral disc prolapse and severe nerve root irritation: sudden onset of low back pain which is so severe that walking is impossible (severe sciatica). Sciatica alone is not absolute indication for referral. Refer if there is difficulty in urinating or defaecating (cauda equina syndrome), or if the condition is progressive or not responding to treatment	**	A27. Red flags of localised diseases of the joints, ligaments and muscles
Cauda equina syndrome: • numbness of the buttocks and perineum (saddle anaesthesia) • bilateral numbness or sciatica in the legs • difficulty in urination or defecation • impaired sexual function	**	A25. Red flags of diseases of the spinal cord and peripheral nerves
Pernicious anaemia: tiredness, lemon-yellow pallor and gradual onset of neurological symptoms (numbness, weakness, confusion)	**/*	A18. Red flags of anaemia

TABLE B28 Red flags of oedema

Symptoms suggestive of:	Priority	For more detail and definitions go to:
Progressive swelling of the soft tissues of the face and neck (angio-oedema) and/or urticaria (nettle rash): refer urgently if there are any features of respiratory distress (itchy throat/wheeze)	***	A41. Red flags of diseases of the skin
Severe chronic heart failure: marked swelling of the ankles and lower legs, disabling breathlessness, cough and exhaustion	**	A14. Red flags of heart failure and arrhythmias
Unexplained oedema (excess tissue fluid, manifesting primarily as ankle swelling extending to >2 cm above the malleoli): possible acute or chronic kidney disease	**	A29. Red flags of diseases of the kidneys

TABLE B28 Continued

Symptoms suggestive of:	Priority	For more detail and definitions go to:
Severe anaemia: extreme tiredness and breathlessness on exertion, excessive bruising, and severe visual disturbances. There may also be features of strain on the cardiovascular system: chest pain on exertion, features of tachycardia and increasing oedema	**	A18. Red flags of anaemia
Oedema, bruising and confusion in someone with known liver disease: suggests liver disease has progressed to a serious stage	**	A8. Red flags of diseases of the liver
Oedema in pregnancy: swelling of ankles is common, but refer if extending >2 cm above the malleoli or if facial oedema is apparent	**	A37. Red flags of pregnancy
Mild chronic heart failure: slight swelling of the ankles, slight breathlessness on exertion and when lying flat, cough, but no palpitations or chest pain	*	A14. Red flags of heart failure and arrhythmias

TABLE B29 Red flags of pain in the bones, joints or muscles

Symptoms suggestive of:	Priority	For more detail and definitions go to:
Limb infarction (suddenly extremely pale, painful, mottled and cold limb): results from a clot in major artery. The life of the limb is threatened	***	A11. Red flags of diseases of the blood vessels
Polymyalgia rheumatica with new onset of one-sided headache: prolonged pain and stiffness of the muscles of the hips and shoulders, associated with malaise and depression. Refer urgently if there is a sudden onset of a severe, one-sided temporal headache or visual disturbances (possible temporal arteritis)	***/**	A28. Red flags of generalised diseases of the joints, ligaments and muscles
Severely compromised circulation to the extremities: pain in the calf which is related to exercise and relieved by rest. Pain in the calf in bed at night relieved by hanging the leg out of bed (i.e. not cramp). Cold, purplish, shiny skin. Areas of blackened skin (gangrene)	**/*	A11. Red flags of diseases of the blood vessels
Deep vein thrombosis: hot, swollen, tender calf; can be accompanied by fever and malaise. Increased risk after air travel and surgery, in pregnancy and cancer, and if on the oral contraceptive pill	**	A11. Red flags of diseases of the blood vessels

TABLE B29 Continued

Symptoms suggestive of:	Priority	For more detail and definitions go to:
Bone pain: characteristically fixed and deep. It may have either an aching or a boring quality. Tenderness on palpation and on percussion. Refer to exclude underlying inflammation or fracture of the bone, both of which result from serious conditions	**/*	A26. Red flags of diseases of the bones
Inflammatory arthritis: symmetrical pain, stiffness and swelling of the joints, or symmetrical stiffness and pain in the sacroiliac joint. May be associated with fever or a sense of malaise	**/*	A28. Red flags of generalised diseases of the joints, ligaments and muscles
Septic or crystal arthritis: a single, hot, swollen and very tender joint. The patient is unwell. Risk of inflammatory damage to the joint	**	A27. Red flags of localised diseases of the joints, ligaments and muscles
Traumatic injury to a muscle or joint (which may require surgical treatment or immobilisation): sudden onset of pain or swelling in a joint (possible haemarthrosis); sudden severe pain and swelling around a joint, with reluctance to move (sprain or strain or possible fracture); locking of the knee joint (meniscal cartilage tear); sudden onset of tender swelling in a muscle (possible haematoma)	**	A27. Red flags of localised diseases of the joints, ligaments and muscles
Intervertebral disc prolapse and severe nerve root irritation: sudden onset of low back pain which is so severe that walking is impossible (severe sciatica). Difficulty urinating or defecating	**	A27. Red flags of localised diseases of the joints, ligaments and muscles
Pubic symphysis pain in pregnancy: refer if the patient is significantly hindered in activities of daily living	**	A37. Red flags of pregnancy
Persistent loin pain (i.e. pain in the flanks either side of the spine between the levels of T11 and L3): pain might be radiating from the kidneys	**	A29. Red flags of diseases of the kidneys
Degenerative arthritis that may benefit from joint replacement: severe disability from long-standing pain and stiffness in the hips, knees or shoulders	*	A28. Red flags of generalised diseases of the joints, ligaments and muscles

TABLE B30 Red flags of palpitations or abnormal pulse rate

Symptoms suggestive of:	Priority	For more detail and definitions go to:
Unstable angina or heart attack: sustained, intense chest pain associated with fear or dread. Palpitations and breathlessness may be present. The patient may vomit or develop a cold sweat *Beware*: in the elderly can present as sudden onset of breathlessness, palpitations or confusion, but without pain	***	A13. Red flags of angina and heart attack
General symptoms of shock: dizziness, fainting and confusion. Rapid pulse of >100 beats/minute. Blood pressure <90/60 mmHg. Cold and clammy extremities. Refer if these symptoms are worsening or sustained (more than a few seconds)	***	A19. Red flags of haemorrhage and shock
A very rapid pulse (140–250 beats/minute): most likely to be supraventricular tachycardia or atrial fibrillation. Refer urgently if ongoing, and as a high priority if has settled down but was the first ever episode	***/**	A14. Red flags of heart failure and arrhythmias
A very slow pulse (40–50 beats/minute) (complete heart block): refer if either of recent onset or if associated with features of shock, such as dizziness, light-headedness or fainting	***/**	A14. Red flags of heart failure and arrhythmias
Severe chronic heart failure: marked swelling of the ankles and lower legs, palpitations, disabling breathlessness, exhaustion	**	A14. Red flags of heart failure and arrhythmias
Complicated pericarditis: palpitations, fever and sharp central chest pain that is worse on leaning forward and lying down. There may be breathlessness due to acute cardiac failure. This is a serious sign	**	A15. Red flags of pericarditis
An irregularly irregular pulse (atrial fibrillation): refer, as there is a risk of embolic stroke as small blood clots can develop in chaotically contracting atria of the heart	**/*	A14. Red flags of heart failure and arrhythmias
Palpitations in pregnancy: refer if it seems that there is any form of arrhythmia in pregnancy. The increased cardiac output in pregnancy can expose previously undiagnosed congenital heart disease	**	A37. Red flags of pregnancy
Hyperthyroidism (symptoms and signs tend to be progressive over the course of a few months). Symptoms: irritability, palpitations, anxiety, sleeplessness, increased appetite, loose stools, weight loss, scanty periods and heat intolerance. Signs: sweaty skin, tremor of the hands, staring eyes and rapid pulse	**/*	A31. Red flags of diseases of the thyroid gland

TABLE B30 Continued

Symptoms suggestive of:	Priority	For more detail and definitions go to:
A pulse that is regular but skips beats at regular intervals (i.e. one out of every 3–5 beats is missing): suggests incomplete heart block. This is an arrhythmia that may precede more serious arrhythmias. Refer for investigation of cause	*	A14. Red flags of heart failure and arrhythmias
Hypothyroidism (symptoms and signs tend to be progressive over the course of a few months). Symptoms: tiredness, depression, weight gain, heavy periods, constipation and cold intolerance. Signs: dry puffy skin, dry and thin hair, slow pulse	*	A26. Red flags of diseases of the thyroid gland

TABLE B31 Red flags of pregnancy and the puerperium

Symptoms suggestive of:	Priority	For more detail and definitions go to:
Pre-eclampsia/HELLP syndromes: headache, abdominal pain, visual disturbance, nausea and vomiting, and oedema (in middle to late pregnancy). These symptoms and signs are serious indicators of the dangerous syndromes of eclampsia and haemolysis/liver abnormalities and low platelets, both of which can threaten the life of the mother and the fetus	***	A37. Red flags of pregnancy
Thromboembolism: pain in the calf, swollen or discoloured leg, or breathlessness with chest pain, or blood in sputum in pregnancy or the puerperium. These symptoms and signs are serious at all times, but are listed here as they are more likely to develop in pregnancy and the puerperium, as there is an increased tendency for the blood to form clots at these stages	***	A37. Red flags of pregnancy
Abdominal pain: refer any episode of sustained abdominal pain in pregnancy as an emergency, particularly if any signs of shock are apparent (low blood pressure, fainting, rapid pulse), as internal bleeding may not be immediately apparent. Abdominal pain may be the first sign of pre-eclampsia. Periodic mild cramping sensations in later pregnancy (lasting no more than a few seconds) are likely to be Braxton Hicks contractions, but if becoming regular and intensifying, beware that these might signify premature labour (if before week 36 of pregnancy) or labour	***	A37. Red flags of pregnancy

TABLE B31 Continued

Symptoms suggestive of:	Priority	For more detail and definitions go to:
Bleeding: refer any episode of vaginal bleeding in pregnancy. Refer as an emergency if any signs of shock are apparent (low blood pressure, fainting, rapid pulse), as internal bleeding may not be immediately apparent	***/**	A37. Red flags of pregnancy
Post-natal psychosis: delusional or paranoid ideas and hallucinations are key features. This condition is associated with a high risk of suicide or harm to the baby	***/**	A38. Red flags of the puerperium
Nausea and vomiting with dehydration for >1 day in pregnancy	**	A37. Red flags of pregnancy
Moderate to severe pregnancy-induced hypertension: refer as a high priority if the diastolic pressure is >100 mmHg or if the systolic pressure is >140 mmHg	**	A37. Red flags of pregnancy
Mild pregnancy-induced hypertension: refer for assessment if the diastolic pressure is 90–99 mmHg and the systolic pressure is <140 mmHg	**	A37. Red flags of pregnancy
Fever with rash in the first trimester of pregnancy: refer suspected rubella or chickenpox so that health of the embryo/fetus can be monitored	**	A37. Red flags of pregnancy
Fever with rash in the last trimester of pregnancy: refer if chickenpox or shingles is suspected, as there is a risk of fatal fetal varicella infection	**	A37. Red flags of pregnancy
Offensive, fishy, watery discharge: possible bacterial vaginosis; there is an increased risk of stillbirth and premature labour	**	A35. Red flags of sexually transmitted diseases
Any watery vaginal leakage in middle to late pregnancy: this is amniotic fluid until proved otherwise	**	A37. Red flags of pregnancy
Fever in the puerperium: refer any case of fever developing in the first 2 weeks of the puerperium (temperature >38°C for >24 hours) as there is a risk this could result from uterine infection	**	A38. Red flags of the puerperium
Mastitis when breastfeeding if not responding to treatment in 2 days, or if there are features of an abscess: mastitis is very debilitating, and if not settling may need antibiotic treatment	**/*	A38. Red flags of the puerperium
Insufficient breast milk or sore nipples: if the mother is considering stopping breastfeeding because of insufficient milk or soreness, refer to the midwife, health visitor or breastfeeding counsellor for breastfeeding advice; the problem may be in the technique, and not a true reflection of low milk production	**/*	A38. Red flags of the puerperium

TABLE B31 Continued

Symptoms suggestive of:	Priority	For more detail and definitions go to:
Post-natal depression lasting for >3 weeks and not responding to your treatment: refer straight away if the woman is experiencing suicidal ideas, or if you believe the health of the baby to be at risk	**/*	A38. Red flags of the puerperium
Itching (severe), especially of the palms and soles in pregnancy: may result from cholestasis (build up of bile salts); refer, as there is a theoretical risk to the health of the fetus if levels rise too high	**	A41. Red flags of diseases of the skin
Oedema in pregnancy: refer all but mild ankle swelling; may result from a kidney or heart problem	*	A37. Red flags of pregnancy
Pubic symphysis pain in pregnancy: refer if the patient is significantly hindered in activities of daily living, as the prescription of a pelvic brace can be a great help	*	A37. Red flags of pregnancy
Anaemia in pregnancy: the risks of bleeding during labour are higher in women with anaemia, so refer for assessment and advice about treatment	*	A37. Red flags of pregnancy
Outbreak of genital herpes in the last trimester of pregnancy: may be an indication for a Caesarean section to prevent the baby contracting the herpesvirus (can be fatal) as it passes through the birth canal	*	A35. Red flags of sexually transmitted diseases
Potential pregnancy-induced hypertension: refer for assessment if the systolic pressure has risen by 30 mmHg or the diastolic pressure by 15 mmHg above any measurement you have taken previously	*	A37. Red flags of pregnancy

TABLE B32 Red flags of diseases of the skin

Symptoms suggestive of:	Priority	For more detail and definitions go to:
Progressive swelling of the soft tissues of the face and neck (angio-oedema) and/or urticaria (nettle rash): refer urgently if there are any features of respiratory distress (itchy throat, wheeze)	***	A41. Red flags of diseases of the skin
Meningococcal septicaemia: acute onset of a purpuric rash, possibly accompanied by headache, vomiting and fever	***	A11. Red flags of diseases of the blood vessels
Bruising and non-blanching rash, together with a severe headache which develops over the course of a few hours to days with fever: suggests meningococcal meningitis	***	A23. Red flags of headache

TABLE B32 Continued

Symptoms suggestive of:	Priority	For more detail and definitions go to:
Purpura or bruising rash (non-blanching): suggests a bleeding disorder or vasculitis. Refer if unexplained, and as a high priority if extensive or rapidly extending	***/**	A41. Red flags of diseases of the skin
Large areas of redness affecting most (>90%) of the body surface (erythroderma): refer because of the risk of dehydration and loss of essential salts	***/**	A41. Red flags of diseases of the skin
A rapidly enlarging patch(es) of painful, crusting or swollen red skin (impetigo or erysipelas): if spreading, refer as a high priority for antibiotic treatment. Refer with some urgency if this occurs in someone with eczema (possible viral eczema herpeticum)	**	A41. Red flags of diseases of the skin
Early shingles: intense, one-sided pain, with an overlying rash of crops of fluid-filled reddened and crusting blisters. The pain may precede the rash by 1–2 days. The pain and rash correspond in location to a neurological dermatome. Refer for early consideration of antiviral treatment	**	A41. Red flags of diseases of the skin
A rapidly advancing region or line of redness tracking up the skin of a limb (following the pathway of a lymphatic vessel): cellulitis and/or lymphangitis	**	A41. Red flags of diseases of the skin
Any new skin ulcer: refer any break in the skin that is not starting to heal within 3 days, or earlier if the margins of the break are widening, or if there are any signs of infection (pus and offensive smell). Be particularly cautious in elderly people and those with diabetes	**	A41. Red flags of diseases of the skin
Cold, purplish, shiny skin suggesting severely compromised circulation to the extremities: may be associated with pain in the calf which relates to exercise and is relieved by rest. Pain in the calf in bed at night relieved by hanging the leg out of bed (i.e. not cramp). These are serious signs of narrowing of the arteries in the pelvis and legs. Refer as high priority if there are areas of blackened skin (gangrene)	**/*	A11. Red flags of diseases of the blood vessels
Generalised macular rash (flat red spots): refer for notification if you suspect rubella, measles or scarlet fever (rash accompanied by significant fever)	**/*	A41. Red flags of diseases of the skin
Lumps/moles with features suggestive of malignancy: • irregularity of shape or pigmentation • recently changing • tendency to bleed • crusting • >5 mm in diameter • intense black colour	*	A41. Red flags of diseases of the skin

TABLE B32 Continued

Symptoms suggestive of:	Priority	For more detail and definitions go to:
Hirsutism (unexplained hairiness): refer to exclude endocrine disease or polycystic ovary syndrome	*	A41. Red flags of diseases of the skin
Itching (severe), especially of the palms and soles in pregnancy: possible cholestasis; refer, as high levels of bile salts may damage the fetus if prolonged	*	A41. Red flags of diseases of the skin
Generalised itch: refer if cause unknown	*	A41. Red flags of diseases of the skin
Pronounced features of candidal infection (thrush) of the skin or mucous membranes of the mouth: suggests underlying diabetes or immunodeficiency	*	A41. Red flags of diseases of the skin
Vaginal itch, if persisting for >3 weeks: the most common cause is candidiasis (thrush), but this should be self-limiting. If persisting, refer to exclude an underlying cause, such as immunodeficiency, malignancy or lichen sclerosus	*	A35. Red flags of sexually transmitted disease
Anal itch, if persisting for >3 weeks: the most common cause is haemorrhoids with skin tags. If persisting, refer to exclude a serious underlying cause, such as anal carcinoma or lichen sclerosus	*	A41. Red flags of diseases of the skin
Eczema of the nipple region (possible Paget's disease)	*	A39. Red flags of diseases of the breast

TABLE B33 Red flags of disorders of speech

Symptoms suggestive of:	Priority	For more detail and definitions go to:
Persistent loss of ability to speak clearly: might result from a persistent loss of neurological function (other features include loss of vision, unsteadiness, confusion, loss of memory, loss of sensation, or muscle weakness). Most likely cause is stroke (thrombotic or haemorrhagic). Needs referring urgently for rapid access to hospital treatment	***	A22. Red flags of brain haemorrhage, stroke and brain tumour A24. Red flags of dementia, epilepsy and other disorders of the central nervous system
Brief loss of ability to speak clearly: suggests a temporary loss of neurological function (usually <2 hours), such as loss of consciousness, loss of vision, unsteadiness, confusion, loss of memory, loss of sensation or limb weakness. If migraine not previously diagnosed, most likely cause is transient ischaemic attack (TIA)	**	A22. Red flags of brain haemorrhage, stroke and brain tumour A24. Red flags of dementia, epilepsy and other disorders of the central nervous system

TABLE B33 Continued

Symptoms suggestive of:	Priority	For more detail and definitions go to:
Progressive loss of ability to speak clearly: may result from a loss of neurological function that is progressive over the course of days to weeks. This is more suggestive of a brain tumour than a stroke. Could also result from multiple sclerosis or motor neurone disease	**	A22. Red flags of brain haemorrhage, stroke and brain tumour
Unexplained hoarseness lasting for >3 weeks: may be the first symptom of laryngeal or lung cancer (particularly in smokers >50 years old)	*	A17. Red flags of lower respiratory disease

TABLE B34 Red flags of disorders of swallowing

Symptoms suggestive of:	Priority	For more detail and definitions go to:
Difficulty swallowing (dysphagia) that is worse with solids (in particular if progressive over days to weeks): suggests a physical obstruction and, if progressive, oesophageal cancer is a possible diagnosis (weight loss is strongly suggestive of this) Other possible causes are oesophageal stricture, oesophageal web (can form in severe anaemia) and candidiasis of the oesophagus (a feature of AIDS). Neurological disease (e.g. stroke and motor neurone disease) can also cause dysfunctional swallowing, and in this case even swallowing of fluids may be difficult Refer for diagnosis and treatment Discomfort in swallowing that does not affect the eating of solids or drinking is very likely to be benign, and does not merit referral	**/*	A5. Red flags of diseases of the oesophagus
Difficulty swallowing (dysphagia) associated with enlarged lymph nodes in the neck: lymph node enlargement suggests the possibility of cancer or an inflammatory mass in the neck (e.g. tuberculous abscess)	**/*	A5. Red flags of diseases of the oesophagus
Swallowing associated with central chest pain (behind the sternum): may result from oesophageal inflammation, an oesophageal tear or a lodged foreign body (fish bone). Refer if persisting for more than a day, or if getting worse	**	A5. Red flags of diseases of the oesophagus

TABLE B35 Red flags of thirst

Symptoms suggestive of:	Priority	For more detail and definitions go to:
Poorly controlled type 1 diabetes or type 2 diabetes: short history of thirst, weight loss and excessive urination, which is rapidly progressive in severity	***/**	A32. Red flags of diabetes mellitus
Type 2 diabetes: general feeling of unwellness, with thirst and increased need to urinate large amounts of urine. These symptoms develop over the course of weeks to months	**/*	A32. Red flags of diabetes mellitus

TABLE B36 Red flags of urinary disorders

Symptoms suggestive of:	Priority	For more detail and definitions go to:
Poorly controlled type 1 diabetes or type 2 diabetes: short history of thirst, weight loss and excessive urination, which is rapidly progressive in severity	***/**	A32. Red flags of diabetes mellitus
Type 2 diabetes: general feeling of malaise, with thirst and increased need to urinate large amounts of urine. These symptoms develop over the course of weeks to months	**/*	A32. Red flags of diabetes mellitus
Urinary tract infection (cloudy urine, painful urination, low abdominal pain, fever) in someone in one of the following vulnerable groups: • pre-existing disorder of the urinary system • diabetes • pregnancy	**	A30. Red flags of diseases of the ureters, bladder and urethra
Vesicoureteric reflux (VUR) disease in a child: any history of recurrent episodes or a current episode of cloudy urine or burning on urination should be taken seriously in a pre-pubescent child	**/*	A29. Red flags of diseases of the kidneys A30. Red flags of diseases of the ureters, bladder and urethra
Recurrent or persistent urinary tract infection: recurrent episodes of symptoms including some or all of cloudy urine, burning on urination, abdominal discomfort, blood in urine and fever, especially if occurring in men. Need to exclude an underlying cause	**/*	A30. Red flags of diseases of the ureters, bladder and urethra
Acute pyelonephritis: fever, malaise, loin pain and cloudy urine suggest an infection of the kidneys	**	A29. Red flags of diseases of the kidneys A30. Red flags of diseases of the ureters, bladder and urethra

TABLE B36 Continued

Symptoms suggestive of:	Priority	For more detail and definitions go to:
Blood in the urine (haematuria) or sperm (haemospermia): refer all cases in men. Refer in women, except in the case of acute urinary infection	**/*	A30. Red flags of diseases of the ureters, bladder and urethra
Intervertebral disc prolapse and severe nerve root irritation: sudden onset of low back pain which is so severe that walking is impossible (severe sciatica); difficulty urinating or defaecating	**	A27. Red flags of localised diseases of the joints, ligaments and muscles
Cauda equina syndrome: numbness of the buttocks and perineum (saddle anaesthesia), with bilateral numbness or sciatica in the legs. Difficulties in urination or defecation are serious symptoms	**	A25. Red flags of diseases of the spinal cord and peripheral nerves
Moderate prostatic obstruction: enlargement of the prostate gland leads to symptoms such as increasing difficulty urinating and the need to get up at night to urinate (nocturia). Refer to assess severity and to exclude prostate cancer	*	A30. Red flags of diseases of the ureters, bladder and urethra
Bedwetting, if persisting over the age of 5 years: refer to exclude a physical or emotional cause	*	A30. Red flags of diseases of the ureters, bladder and urethra
Incontinence, if unexplained or causing distress: refer for investigations and advice from an incontinence specialist nurse	*	A30. Red flags of diseases of the ureters, bladder and urethra

TABLE B37 Red flags of visual disturbance

Symptoms suggestive of:	Priority	For more detail and definitions go to:
Blurred vision in malignant hypertension: diastolic pressure >120 mmHg, with symptoms including recently worsening headaches, blurred vision and chest pain	***/**	A12. Red flags of hypertension
Blurred vision in pre-eclampsia/HELLP syndromes: headache, abdominal pain, visual disturbance, nausea and vomiting, and oedema (in middle to late pregnancy)	***	A37. Red flags of pregnancy
Sudden blurring of vision with a one-sided headache in an older person: consider temporal arteritis if there is no history of migraine. Refer urgently for steroid treatment, as the risk of blindness and stroke is high	***	A42. Red flags of diseases of the eye

TABLE B37 Continued

Symptoms suggestive of:	Priority	For more detail and definitions go to:
A temporary, persisting or progressive loss of clarity of sight due to brain dysfunction: may result from loss of neurological function in migraine, transient ischaemic attack or stroke. Other symptoms include loss of consciousness, loss of vision, unsteadiness, confusion, loss of memory, loss of sensation or limb weakness. Refer urgently if the loss of neurological function is persisting and as a high priority if temporary	**/***	A22. Red flags of brain haemorrhage, stroke and brain tumour A24. Red flags of dementia, epilepsy and other disorders of the central nervous system
Painless sudden loss of sight: may result from retinal detachment, vitreous detachment or retinal artery thrombosis. Refer as a high priority to the emergency department, as retinal detachment is treatable if caught early	**	A42. Red flags of diseases of the eye
Visual disturbance from the growth of a pituitary tumour: features include progressive headaches, visual disturbance and double vision	**/*	A33. Red flags of other endocrine diseases
Severe anaemia: extreme tiredness and breathlessness on exertion, excessive bruising and severe visual disturbances suggest that the anaemia is very severe. There may also be features of strain on the cardiovascular system: chest pain on exertion, features of tachycardia and increasing oedema	**	A18. Red flags of anaemia
Thyroid eye disease (vision only affected if very advanced). Symptoms: irritability, anxiety, sleeplessness, increased appetite, loose stools, weight loss, scanty periods and heat intolerance. Signs: sweaty skin, tremor of the hands, staring eyes and rapid pulse	**/*	A31. Red flags of diseases of the thyroid gland
Optic neuritis: blurred vision with deep aching pain in the eye. Associated with multiple sclerosis. Refer for diagnosis	**	A42. Red flags of diseases of the eye

TABLE B38 Red flags of vomiting and/or passage of faeces

Symptoms suggestive of:	Priority	For more detail and definitions go to:
Severe headache that develops over the course of a few hours to days with fever, together with either vomiting or neck stiffness: possible acute meningitis or encephalitis	***	A23. Red flags of headache
Meningococcal septicaemia: acute onset of purpuric rash, possibly accompanied by headache, vomiting and fever	***	A11. Red flags of diseases of the blood vessels

TABLE B38 Continued

Symptoms suggestive of:	Priority	For more detail and definitions go to:
Diarrhoea and vomiting associated with features of dehydration	***/**	A6. Red flags of diseases of the stomach
Severe diarrhoea and vomiting if lasting >24 hours in infants or the elderly	***/**	A6. Red flags of diseases of the stomach
Projectile vomiting persisting for >2 days	***/**	A6. Red flags of diseases of the stomach
Vomiting of fresh blood or altered blood (looks like dark gravel or coffee grounds)	***/**	A6. Red flags of diseases of the stomach A8. Red flags of diseases of the liver
Right hypochondriac pain that is very intense and comes in waves: may be associated with fever and vomiting. May be associated with jaundice. This is one of the manifestations of the acute abdomen	***/**	A9. Red flags of diseases of the gallbladder
Addison's disease: increased pigmentation of skin, weight loss, muscle wasting, tiredness, loss of libido, low blood pressure, diarrhoea and vomiting, confusion, collapse with dehydration	***/**	A33. Red flags of other endocrine diseases
Diarrhoea and/or vomiting in an elderly person: treat with caution, as the elderly are prone to dehydration, and diarrhoea and vomiting may be presenting features of more serious underlying disease	**	A2. Red flags of infectious diseases: vulnerable groups
Diarrhoea and/or vomiting in infants (especially if <3 months old): treat with caution, as infants are prone to dehydration, and diarrhoea and vomiting may be presenting features of more serious underlying disease	**	A2. Red flags of infectious diseases: vulnerable groups
Diarrhoea and/or vomiting in an immunocompromised person: treat with caution; diarrhoea and vomiting may be features of a serious infection in people who are immunocompromised	**	A2. Red flags of infectious diseases: vulnerable groups
Diarrhoea and vomiting if continuing for >5 days in otherwise healthy adults: most mild infections should have settled down in 2–3 days; needs further investigation	**	A6. Red flags of diseases of the stomach
Diarrhoea with mucus or gripy pain if not responding to treatment within a week: possible inflammatory bowel disease or parasitic infection	**	A10. Red flags of diseases of the small and large intestines
Altered bowel habit lasting for >3 weeks in a patient >50 years old	**/*	A10. Red flags of diseases of the small and large intestines

TABLE B38 Continued

Symptoms suggestive of:	Priority	For more detail and definitions go to:
Infectious bloody diarrhoea or food poisoning: an episode of diarrhoea and vomiting in which food is suspected as the origin or in which blood appears in the stools: these are notifiable diseases	**	A10. Red flags of diseases of the small and large intestines
Nausea and vomiting with dehydration (dry skin, dry mouth, low blood pressure, low skin turgor) for >1 day in pregnancy: patient may need fluid replacement	**	A37. Red flags of pregnancy
Cauda equina syndrome: numbness of the buttocks and perineum (saddle anaesthesia), with bilateral numbness or sciatica in the legs; difficulty in urination or defecation are serious symptoms	**	A25 Red flags of diseases of the spinal cord and peripheral nerves
Soiling of stool or anal discharge (in underwear or bed) in a previously continent child or adult: may signify constipation in both children and the elderly, and also emotional distress in a child. In adults, anal discharge may be a sign of anorectal carcinoma	*	A10. Red flags of diseases of the small and large intestines
Slow increase in intracranial pressure: progressive headaches and vomiting over a timescale of a few weeks to months. The headaches are worse in the morning, and the vomiting may be effortless. Blurring of vision and confusion may be additional symptoms	**	A21. Red flags of raised intracranial pressure
Vertigo (dizziness) in young person: usually due to benign labyrinthitis and will settle down. Refer if lasting for >6 weeks, or if so severe as to be causing recurrent vomiting. Refer if patient is at increased risk of thromboembolic disease (e.g. in pregnancy) so that the possibility of stroke can be excluded	**/*	A43. Red flags of diseases of the ear
Vertigo (dizziness) in an older person (>45 years old): refer for medical assessment straightaway. Although still more likely to be a result of inner ear disease, stroke is also a possible cause in this age group	**	A43. Red flags of diseases of the ear
Hyperthyroidism. Symptoms: irritability, anxiety, sleeplessness, increased appetite, loose stools, weight loss, scanty periods and heat intolerance. Signs: sweaty skin, tremor of the hands, staring eyes and rapid pulse	**/*	A31. Red flags of diseases of the thyroid gland

TABLE B39 Red flags of weakness/paralysis

Symptoms suggestive of:	Priority	For more detail and definitions go to:
Any sudden or gradual onset of muscle weakness that might be affecting muscles of respiration: refer urgently	***	A25. Red flags of diseases of the spinal cord and peripheral nerves
Addison's disease: increased pigmentation of skin, weight loss, muscle wasting, tiredness, loss of libido, low blood pressure, diarrhoea and vomiting, confusion, collapse with dehydration	***/**	A33. Red flags of other endocrine diseases
Weakness that results from a temporary, progressive or persisting loss of neurological function: suggested by accompanying symptoms such as loss of consciousness, loss of vision, unsteadiness, confusion, loss of memory or loss of sensation. Possible stroke, transient ischaemic attack or brain tumour. Refer urgently if persisting and high priority if temporary	**/***	A22. Red flags of brain haemorrhage, stroke and brain tumour A24. Red flags of dementia, epilepsy and other disorders of the central nervous system
Any sudden or gradual onset of muscle weakness that can be objectively assessed (i.e. not just the patient's perception of weakness): refer to exclude serious muscular or neurological condition (e.g. myasthenia gravis, polymyositis, peripheral neuropathy or mononeuropathy, motor neurone disease)	**/*	A25. Red flags of diseases of the spinal cord and peripheral nerves
Cauda equina syndrome: numbness of the buttocks and perineum (saddle anaesthesia), with bilateral numbness, weakness or sciatica in the legs. Difficulty in urination or defecation are serious symptoms	**	A25. Red flags of diseases of the spinal cord and peripheral nerves
Bell's palsy: sudden onset of facial weakness; almost always unilateral. Refer for same-day treatment with antiviral and steroid medication	**	A25. Red flags of diseases of the spinal cord and peripheral nerves
Cushing's syndrome: weight gain, weakness and wasting of limb muscles, stretch marks and bruises. Mood changes, hypertension, red cheeks, acne	*	A33. Red flags of other endocrine diseases

TABLE B40 Red flags of weight loss or weight gain

Symptoms suggestive of:	Priority	For more detail and definitions go to:
Progressive unexplained symptoms over weeks to months (e.g. weight loss, recurrent sweats, fevers, poor appetite): may be cancer, HIV or tuberculosis	**/*	A1. Red flags of cancer
Malabsorption syndrome (loose, pale stools and malnutrition): weight loss, thin hair, dry skin, cracked lips and peeled tongue. Will present as failure to thrive in children. Causes include coeliac disease and chronic pancreatitis	**/*	A7. Red flags of diseases of the pancreas A10. Red flags of diseases of the small and large intestines
Tuberculosis infection: chronic productive cough, weight loss, night sweats, blood in sputum for >2 weeks	**	A17. Red flags of lower respiratory disease
Hyperthyroidism (symptoms and signs tend to be progressive over the course of a few months). Symptoms: irritability, anxiety, sleeplessness, increased appetite, loose stools, weight loss, scanty periods and heat intolerance. Signs: sweaty skin, tremor of the hands, staring eyes and rapid pulse	**/*	A31. Red flags of diseases of the thyroid gland
Severe disturbance of body image: if not responding to your treatment, and resulting in features of progressive anorexia nervosa or bulimia nervosa (e.g. progressive weight loss, secondary amenorrhoea, or repeated compulsion to bring about vomiting)	*	A44. Red flags of mental health disorders
Hypothyroidism (symptoms and signs tend to be progressive over the course of a few months). Symptoms: tiredness, depression, weight gain, heavy periods, constipation and cold intolerance. Signs: dry puffy skin, dry and thin hair, slow pulse	*	A31. Red flags of diseases of the thyroid gland
Cushing's syndrome: weight gain, weakness and wasting of limb muscles, stretch marks and bruises. Mood changes, hypertension, red cheeks, acne	*	A33. Red flags of other endocrine diseases

CHAPTER 4

C TABLES: RED FLAGS REQUIRING URGENT REFERRAL

INTRODUCTION

The C tables present 12 categories of red flag syndromes in which an urgent or high priority response is required from the therapist.

Each C table is accompanied with a brief guide to first-aid management. This guidance is intended for the use of qualified first aiders, or for the purposes of the training of therapists in first aid.

The red flags are referenced to those found in the A tables in Chapter 2 so that the reader can access more information about these symptoms and signs and their underlying medical conditions.

The order of the C tables can be found in the contents pages of this text.

TABLE C1 Red flags of acute abdominal pain

Symptoms suggestive of:	Priority	For more detail and definitions go to:
Severe abdominal pain with collapse ('the acute abdomen'): the pain can be constant or colicky (coming in waves)	***/**	A6. Red flags of diseases of the stomach A10. Red flags of diseases of the small and large intestines
Acute pancreatitis: presents as the acute abdomen, with severe central abdominal and back pain, vomiting and dehydration	***/**	A7. Red flags of diseases of the pancreas
Obstructed gallstone: right hypochondriac pain (pain under the right ribs) which is very intense and comes in waves. May be associated with fever and vomiting, and jaundice	***/**	A9. Red flags of diseases of the gallbladder
Obstructed kidney stone: acute loin pain (pain in the flanks radiating round to pubic region) which comes in waves. May be associated vomiting, agitation and collapse	***	A30. Red flags of diseases of the ureters, bladder and urethra

TABLE C1 Continued

Symptoms suggestive of:	Priority	For more detail and definitions go to:
Acute testicular pain (torsion of testis): radiates to groin, scrotum or lower abdomen. May be associated vomiting and collapse	***/**	A36. Red flags of structural disorders of the reproductive system
Pelvic inflammatory disease (acute form): lower abdominal pain with collapse and fever	***	A35. Red flags of sexually transmitted diseases
Ruptured aortic aneurysm: acute abdominal or back pain with collapse and features of shock	***	A11. Red flags of diseases of the blood vessels
Sustained severe abdominal pain in pregnancy: may be ruptured ectopic pregnancy, placental abruption, pre-eclampsia or premature labour	***/**	A37. Red flags of pregnancy
Premature labour: periodic mild cramping sensations in later pregnancy (lasting no more than a few seconds) are likely to be Braxton Hicks contractions, but if becoming regular and intensifying, beware that these might signify premature labour (by definition, before week 36 of pregnancy)	***/**	A37. Red flags of pregnancy
Pre-eclampsia/HELLP (hemolysis, elevated liver enzymes, low platelet count) syndromes in pregnancy: headache, abdominal or epigastric pain, visual disturbance, nausea and vomiting and oedema (in middle to late pregnancy)	***/**	A37. Red flags of pregnancy

Notes

– All these syndromes involve severe abdominal, pelvic or loin pain with 'collapse' (i.e. inability to carry out normal activities). Patients may lie still, or may be restless with pain, depending on the cause. 'Collapse' is a potentially confusing medical term, as it may conjure up ideas of a patient in a heap on the floor. In a medical context, the term is used simply to suggest that the patient is unable to carry out daily activities. A patient so distracted by abdominal pain that their pain is all they can attend to at the time (and usually pain of this magnitude would cause them to lie down) would be considered to have abdominal pain with collapse, even if they are fully conscious.

– Rigidity, guarding and rebound tenderness are serious signs found on abdominal examination. Rigidity means that the abdominal muscles are in reflex spasm because of pain. Guarding describes a region of localised muscle spasm overlying a region of inflammation. Rebound tenderness describes the patient's experience of discomfort when the pressure from an examining hand on the abdomen is released. Causes of these signs on examination of the abdomen include perforated viscus, peritonitis, appendicitis, bowel obstruction, ruptured aortic aneurysm, acute pancreatitis, bowel infarction and ectopic pregnancy.

First-aid measures for acute abdominal pain and collapse

- Call for medical assistance.
- Ensure the patient is kept comfortable and warm.
- Ensure the patient has no food or drink.
- If there are features of shock (see **C3**), ensure the patient is lying down.
- Place in the recovery position only if there is loss of consciousness.

TABLE C2 Red flags of bone marrow failure

Symptoms suggestive of:	Priority	For more detail and definitions go to:
Bone marrow failure: symptoms of progressive anaemia, recurrent progressive infections, and progressive bruising, purpura and bleeding	***/**	A1. Red flags of cancer A20. Red flags of leukaemia and lymphoma

Notes

– Failure of the bone marrow to produce the three cellular components of the blood leads to anaemia (due to low red blood cell count), bleeding (due to low platelet count) and intractable infections (due to low lymphocyte count). The patient will be pale, exhausted, may have purpura (dark purple macules on the skin), nosebleeds and fever.

– Bone marrow failure most commonly results from advanced secondary cancer or leukaemia or lymphoma. It can also be the result of reactions to drug therapy, including chemotherapy. The patient is at risk of succumbing to devastating bleeding or overwhelming infections and needs urgent medical assessment.

First-aid measures for bone marrow failure

- Call for medical assistance.
- Ensure the patient is kept comfortable and warm.
- Stem any sources of blood loss.
- If there are features of shock (see **C3**), ensure the patient is lying down.
- Place in the recovery position only if there is loss of consciousness.

TABLE C3 Red flags of blood loss and shock

Symptoms suggestive of:	Priority	For more detail and definitions go to:
Continuing blood loss: any situation in which significant bleeding is continuing for more than a few minutes without any signs of abating (e.g. nosebleed), except within the context of menstruation, is potentially serious	***/**	A19. Red flags of haemorrhage and shock
Vomiting of fresh blood or altered blood (haematemesis): if blood is altered, it looks like dark gravel or coffee grounds in the vomit. Refer urgently if any signs of shock (see **A19.3**) are present	***/**	A6. Red flags of diseases of the stomach A8. Red flags of diseases of the liver

TABLE C3 Continued

Symptoms suggestive of:	Priority	For more detail and definitions go to:
Altered blood in stools (melaena): stools look like black tar. Suggests large amount of bleeding from stomach. Refer urgently if any signs of shock (see **A19.3**) are present	***/**	A6. Red flags of diseases of the stomach
Bleeding: refer any episode of vaginal bleeding in pregnancy as an emergency if any signs of shock (see **A19.3**) are apparent	***/**	A37. Red flags of pregnancy
Post-partum (after delivery of baby) haemorrhage with a bleed of >500 ml or the symptoms of shock (see **A19.3**)	***/**	A38. Red flags of the puerperium
A very rapid pulse of 140–250 beats/minute: most likely to be supraventricular tachycardia or atrial fibrillation. Refer urgently if ongoing, and as a high priority if has settled down but was first ever episode	***/**	A14. Red flags of heart failure and arrhythmias
A very slow pulse of 40–50 beats/minute (complete heart block): refer if either of recent onset or if associated with features of shock (see **A19.3**), such as dizziness, light-headedness or fainting	***/**	A14. Red flags of heart failure and arrhythmias

Notes

– Bleeding becomes an emergency situation if the blood loss is so severe as to threaten the development of the syndrome of shock (see **A19.3**). Shock is defined as any situation in which the circulation of the blood is not sufficient to meet bodily demands. The symptoms and signs of shock include feeling dizzy or faint with low blood pressure and collapse. As it is impossible to assess the exact volume of internal bleeding, refer all significant episodes of internal bleeding (e.g. in vomit, in stools, in pregnancy) as an emergency.

– If blood loss is the cause of shock, this is a form of hypovolaemic shock. In this case, the body responds by releasing the hormone adrenaline. This causes constriction of blood vessels and raises the heart rate. The patient will, therefore, have cold extremities and a racing pulse. The adrenaline may raise the blood pressure back to the normal range, and so the raised heart rate may be the cardinal red flag sign.

– Infection and allergic reaction can also cause shock, because in extreme cases the release of inflammatory chemicals can lead to widespread dilatation of the blood vessels and so cause a profound drop in blood pressure. The blood volume is normal in this case. The patient may seem warm and flushed, rather than cold, but the pulse rate will be increased, as it is with blood loss.

– Shock can also result from poor pumping efficiency of the heart (cardiogenic shock). This might occur after a heart attack, in heart failure or during an arrhythmia. In this case the prime features are faintness/collapse and low blood pressure.

– Simple fainting also results from a sudden drop in blood pressure, this time because of the release of hormones that cause a reduction in heart rate, and therefore a drop in blood pressure. Simple fainting is always characterised by a return to consciousness and normalisation of the pulse and blood pressure within a few seconds to minutes. Emotional factors and/or low blood sugar can trigger fainting. There is no need to refer a single episode of simple fainting. If the loss of consciousness is for more than a few seconds, then this is not characteristic of a faint and merits further investigations.

First-aid measures for blood loss and shock

● Call for medical assistance.
● Ensure the patient is kept comfortable and warm.
● Stem any sources of external blood loss by firm pressure, and raise any limbs which are bleeding.
● If there are features of shock (low blood pressure and feelings of faintness), first check there are no breathing difficulties. If not, then ensure the patient is lying down.
● Place in recovery position if there is possibility of vomiting or if there is loss of consciousness.
● Continue to check airway, breathing and circulation (ABC). If no breathing, then call the emergency services and be prepared to perform cardiopulmonary resuscitation (CPR). (NB: If there are features of shock and breathing difficulty, this suggests possible anaphylaxis. Treat as described below under 'acute difficulty in breathing'.)

TABLE C4 Red flags of acute difficulty in breathing

Symptoms suggestive of:	Priority	For more detail and definitions go to:
Severe asthma. At least two of the following: rapidly worsening breathlessness, >30 respirations/minute (or more if a child[1]), heart rate >110 beats/minute, reluctance to talk because of breathlessness, need to sit upright and still to assist breathing. Cyanosis is a very serious sign	***	A17. Red flags of lower respiratory disease
Infection of the lower respiratory tract (pneumonia): cough, fever, malaise, >30 respirations/minute (or more if a child[1]), heart rate >110 beats/minute, reluctance to talk because of breathlessness, need to sit upright and still to assist breathing. Cyanosis is a very serious sign	***/**	A17. Red flags of lower respiratory disease
Central cyanosis: cyanosis seen on the tongue suggests poor oxygenation of the blood and merits urgent referral if of recent onset in an unwell person	***	A17. Red flags of lower respiratory disease
Pulmonary embolism: sudden onset of pleurisy (chest pain exacerbated by breathing in), with breathlessness, cyanosis, collapse, and blood in sputum	***	A17. Red flags of lower respiratory disease
Sudden lung collapse (pneumothorax): onset of severe breathlessness, may be some pleurisy (chest pain exacerbated by breathing in), and collapse if very severe	***	A17. Red flags of lower respiratory disease
Stridor (harsh noisy breathing heard on both the inbreath and outbreath): suggests obstruction to upper airway. Patient will want to sit upright and still. Do not ask to examine the tongue	***/**	A16. Red flags of upper respiratory disease
A single, grossly enlarged tonsil and difficulty in breathing: if the patient is unwell and feverish and has foul-smelling breath, this suggests quinsy. This is a surgical emergency, as breathing may be compromised	***/**	A16. Red flags of upper respiratory disease

TABLE C4 Continued

Symptoms suggestive of:	Priority	For more detail and definitions go to:
Acute heart failure: sudden onset of disabling breathlessness and watery cough	***	A14. Red flags of heart failure and arrhythmias
Any sudden or gradual onset of muscle weakness that might be affecting muscles of respiration: needs to be referred urgently as the condition may progress to respiratory failure	***	A25. Red flags of diseases of the spinal cord and peripheral nerves

¹Categorisation of respiratory rate in adults

– Normal respiratory rate in an adult: 10–20 breaths/minute (one breath is one inhalation and exhalation).
– Moderate breathlessness in an adult: >30 breaths/minute.
– Severe breathlessness in an adult: >60 breaths/minute.

Categorisation of respiratory rate in children

The normal range for respiratory rate in children varies according to age.

The following rates indicate moderate to severe breathlessness:

newborn (0–3 months)	>60 breaths/minute
infant (3 months to 2 years)	>50 breaths/minute
young child (2–8 years)	>40 breaths/minute
older child to adult	>30 breaths/minute.

Notes

– Most situations in which the act of respiration is becoming insufficient to meet bodily requirements is characterised by rapid respirations (especially if >30 breaths/minute in adults), a sense of panic and, if severe, cyanosis (bluish coloration to the lips and tongue). The rapid respirations are a reflex response mediated by the respiratory centre in the brain stem which detect rising levels of carbon dioxide in the blood. Cyanosis is the visible sign that the haemoglobin in the blood is under-oxygenated. This pigment changes from red to purplish blue when the saturation of oxygen falls to less than 85%. In health, the saturation of oxygen of the blood is greater than 98%.

– In the cases of acute muscle weakness, or suppression of respiration resulting from stroke or drug intoxication, there can be insufficient respiration but without associated breathlessness. In this case, the red flag signs are shallow breathing, cyanosis and drowsiness. This is an emergency situation.

– Stridor is a harsh inspiratory and expiratory noise which comes from the upper airways, and indicates severe potential obstruction (either due to a swelling or a foreign body). A person in this situation will want to sit still and upright. The patient should not be asked to show his or her tongue in this situation, as this may worsen the obstruction.

First-aid measures for acute difficulty in breathing

- Ensure the patient is kept calm and upright. Increase access to fresh air if possible. Steam may help (i.e. take patient to be near a running shower) if infection is a possible cause.
- If the patient is asthmatic, ensure they take four puffs of reliever (blue inhaler) medication as soon as possible, ideally via a spacer. Repeat this every 5 minutes until help arrives, or until the attack is relieved.
- Do not ask to examine the tongue.
- If features of shock are present (low blood pressure, and dizziness or fainting) together with difficulty breathing, this may suggest anaphylaxis. Check to see if the patient is carrying an 'epipen' and, if so, ensure that a metered dose of adrenaline is administered if at all possible.
- In all cases, if the person loses consciousness and respiration is ineffective, call for help, ensure the airway is open and commence cardiopulmonary resuscitation (CPR).

TABLE C5 Red flags of chest pain

Symptoms suggestive of:	Priority	For more detail and definitions go to:
Unstable angina or heart attack: sustained intense chest pain associated with fear or dread. Palpitations and breathlessness may be present. The patient may vomit or develop a cold sweat. Beware: in the elderly can present as sudden onset of breathlessness, palpitations or confusion, but without pain	***	A13. Red flags of angina and heart attack
Complicated pericarditis: sharp central chest pain which is worse on leaning forward and lying down. Fever. Associated palpitations and breathlessness are more serious features	***/**	A15. Red flags of pericarditis
Dissecting aortic aneurysm: sudden onset of tearing chest pain with radiation to back. Features of shock may be present (faintness, low blood pressure, rapid pulse)	***	A13. Red flags of angina and heart attack
Pulmonary embolism: sudden onset of pleurisy (chest pain related to breathing in) with breathlessness, cyanosis, collapse and blood in sputum	***	A17. Red flags of lower respiratory disease
Sudden lung collapse (pneumothorax): breathlessness, may be some pleurisy, and collapse if very severe	***	A17. Red flags of lower respiratory disease

Notes

- Causes of chest pain which merit emergency referral include myocardial ischaemia, pneumonia with pleurisy, dissecting aortic aneurysm, pulmonary embolus and pneumothorax.
- Serious chest pain of cardiac origin is characteristically heavy and radiates to the throat and upper arms. The patient may experience dread, breathlessness and palpitations. Serious chest pain of respiratory origin will be associated with breathing and breathlessness. The patient will be anxious.

– Chest pain is a common aspect of a panic attack. In this case, the pain may be more to one side and be described as stabbing in nature. It is more likely to occur for the first time in a young person. Breathlessness and tingling of the fingers may also be features. Although the best response is reassurance only, if you have any doubt, refer as if of cardiac origin.

First-aid measures for acute chest pain

- Call for medical assistance.
- Ensure the patient is kept comfortable, upright and warm.
- If you suspect that the pain is of cardiac origin, first check that the patient is not pregnant, on anticoagulant medication, has no history of peptic ulcer disease, and no known allergy to aspirin or aspirin-induced asthma. If not, administer 300 mg (1 tablet) of soluble aspirin as soon as possible.
- If the patient loses consciousness, check airway, breathing and circulation (ABC). If breathing, keep in the recovery position. If not breathing, call emergency services and be prepared to perform cardiopulmonary resuscitation (CPR).

TABLE C6 Red flags of dehydration

Symptoms suggestive of:	Priority	For more detail and definitions go to:
Dehydration in an infant: dry mouth and skin, loss of skin turgor (firmness), drowsiness, sunken fontanelle (soft spot in the region of acupoint Du24) and dry nappies	***/**	A3. Red flags of infectious diseases: fever, dehydration and confusion
Severe diarrhoea and vomiting if lasting >24 hours in infants, pregnancy or the elderly	***/**	A6. Red flags of diseases of the stomach
Projectile vomiting persisting for >2 days, or any projectile vomiting in a newborn: suggests obstruction to the outflow of the stomach and high risk of salt/fluid imbalance	***/**	A6. Red flags of diseases of the stomach
Poorly controlled type 1 diabetes or type 2 diabetes: short history of thirst, weight loss and excessive urination which is rapidly progressive in severity. Can progress to confusion/coma with dehydration (due to hyperglycaemia)	***/**	A32. Red flags of diabetes mellitus
Addison's disease: increased pigmentation of skin, weight loss, muscle wasting, tiredness, loss of libido, low blood pressure, diarrhoea and vomiting, confusion, collapse with dehydration	***/**	A33. Red flags of other endocrine diseases

Notes

– Possible causes of dehydration include excess climatic heat, prolonged fever, diarrhoea and vomiting, hyperglycaemia in diabetes mellitus and poor intake of fluids in a frail person or infant. Dehydration leads to concentration of the salts in the blood, ineffective removal of toxins by the kidneys and poor circulation to the brain and kidneys.

– Features of dehydration include dry mouth and skin, low blood pressure, weakness in adults, concentrated urine, floppiness, sunken eyes and fontanelle in infants, and loss of consciousness.

– Dehydration requires a rapid response in infants, in pregnancy and the elderly – these groups are more vulnerable to kidney damage and circulatory collapse.

First-aid measures for dehydration

- Call for medical assistance.
- Ensure the patient is kept comfortable and warm, and administer fluids by mouth (warm water) if possible.
- If the patient loses consciousness, check airway, breathing and circulation (ABC). If breathing, keep in the recovery position. If not breathing, call emergency services and be prepared to perform cardiopulmonary resuscitation (CPR).

TABLE C7 Red flags of weakness or loss of consciousness

Symptoms suggestive of:	Priority	For more detail and definitions go to:
Cardiac arrest: collapse with no palpable pulse	***	A14. Red flags of heart failure and arrhythmias
Rapid increase in intracranial pressure (intracranial haemorrhage): headache followed by a rapid deterioration of consciousness leading to coma. Irregular breathing patterns and pinpoint pupils are a very serious sign. May be spontaneous or may result from a head injury	***	A21. Red flags of raised intracranial pressure A22. Red flags of brain haemorrhage, stroke and brain tumour
A persisting loss of neurological function, such as loss of consciousness, loss of vision, unsteadiness, confusion, loss of memory, loss of sensation or muscle weakness	***	A22. Red flags of brain haemorrhage, stroke and brain tumour
Sudden lung collapse (pneumothorax): onset of severe breathlessness, may be some pleurisy (chest pain on breathing in) and collapse if very severe	***	A17. Red flags of lower respiratory disease
Pulmonary embolism: sudden onset of pleurisy (chest pain on breathing in) with breathlessness, cyanosis, collapse	***	A17. Red flags of lower respiratory disease
A severe headache that develops over the course of a few hours to days with fever, together with either vomiting or neck stiffness. The patient may become drowsy or unconscious. Suggests acute meningitis or encephalitis	***	A23. Red flags of headache
Confusion/coma with dehydration (hyperglycaemia)	***	A32. Red flags of diabetes mellitus
Hypoglycaemia (due to effects of insulin or antidiabetic medication in excess of bodily requirements): agitation, sweating, dilated pupils, confusion and coma	***	A32. Red flags of diabetes mellitus
General symptoms of shock: dizziness, fainting and confusion. Rapid pulse of >100 beats/minute. Blood pressure <90/60 mmHg. Cold and clammy extremities. Refer if symptoms are worsening or sustained (more than a few seconds)	***	A19. Red flags of haemorrhage and shock

TABLE C7 Continued

Symptoms suggestive of:	Priority	For more detail and definitions go to:
Addison's disease: increased pigmentation of skin, weight loss, muscle wasting, tiredness, loss of libido, low blood pressure, diarrhoea and vomiting, confusion, collapse, dehydration	***/**	A33. Red flags of other endocrine diseases
Febrile convulsion in child: ongoing	***	A3. Red flags of infectious diseases: fever, dehydration and confusion
First ever epileptic seizure. Generalised tonic–clonic seizure: convulsions, loss of consciousness, bitten tongue, emptying of bladder and/or bowels. This is an emergency if the fit does not settle down within 2 minutes. Refer as a high priority if the fit has settled down	***	A23. Red flags of dementia, epilepsy and other disorders of the central nervous system
Simple fainting: dizziness, temporary collapse (no more than a few seconds) and temporary confusion. Normal or slowed pulse rate. Blood pressure <90/60 mmHg. Cold and clammy extremities. Patient starts to recover in seconds to a minute. No need to refer	–	A19. Red flags of haemorrhage and shock

Notes

- Possible causes of loss of consciousness include fainting, cardiac arrest, respiratory arrest, brain haemorrhage or infarction (stroke), drug intoxication, endocrine disorder (diabetes or Addison's disease), brain infection (e.g. meningitis) and epileptic fit.
- All cases of continued measurable weakness (i.e a paralysis) or loss of consciousness are emergencies unless the cause is known.
- Anyone who has recovered from an episode of paralysis or loss of consciousness needs to be considered for high-priority referral for investigation if the cause is unknown.

First-aid measures for loss of consciousness

- Call for medical assistance.
- If still unconscious, check the patient is in a safe and warm setting, and place in the recovery position with the airway held open.
- Continue to check airway, breathing and circulation (ABC). If not breathing, call emergency services and be prepared to perform cardiopulmonary resuscitation (CPR).
- If recovering from an episode of paralysis or loss of consciousness, ensure the patient is kept safe until fully recovered. If you do not know cause, ensure medical opinion is sought. Advise the patient not to drive and not to be alone until he or she has been seen by a doctor.

TABLE C8 Red flags of confusion or altered mental state

Symptoms suggestive of:	Priority	For more detail and definitions go to:
A persisting loss of neurological function, such as loss of consciousness, loss of vision, unsteadiness, confusion, loss of memory, loss of sensation or muscle weakness	***	A22. Red flags of brain haemorrhage, stroke and brain tumour
Organic mental health disorder (a mental health condition due to an underlying gross physical cause): acute confusion, agitation, deterioration in intellectual skills, loss of ability to care for self. These symptoms suggest organic brain disorder such as metabolic disease, drug intoxication, brain damage or dementia	***/**	A44. Red flags of mental health disorders
Unusual drowsiness present in infants (especially if <3 months old): may signify underlying serious illness	***/**	A2. Red flags of infectious diseases: vulnerable groups
Poorly controlled type 1 diabetes or type 2 diabetes: short history of thirst, weight loss and excessive urination which is rapidly progressive in severity. Can progress to confusion/coma with dehydration (due to hyperglycaemia)	***/**	A32. Red flags of diabetes mellitus
Hypoglycaemia (due to effects of insulin or antidiabetic medication in excess of bodily requirements): agitation, sweating, dilated pupils, confusion and coma	***	A32. Red flags of diabetes mellitus
Hyperthyroidism: irritability, anxiety, confusional state, sleeplessness, increased appetite, loose stools, weight loss, scanty periods and heat intolerance. Signs: sweaty skin, tremor of the hands, staring eyes and rapid pulse	**/*	A31. Red flags of diseases of the thyroid gland
Hallucinations, delusions or other evidence of thought disorder together with evidence of deteriorating self-care and personality change: all features of a psychosis such as schizophrenia. Suicide risk is high. Refer urgently if behaviour is posing risk to the patient or others	***/**	A44. Red flags of mental health disorders
Mania: increasing agitation, grandiosity, pressure of speech and sleeplessness, with delusional thinking. All features of bipolar disorder, a form of psychosis which carries a high risk of behaviour that can be both socially and physically damaging to the patient. Suicide risk is high. Refer urgently if behaviour is posing risk to the patient or others	***/**	A44. Red flags of mental health disorders
Post-natal psychosis: delusional or paranoid ideas and hallucinations are key features. This condition is associated with a high risk of suicide or harm to the baby	***/**	A38. Red flags of the puerperium

TABLE C8 Continued

Symptoms suggestive of:	Priority	For more detail and definitions go to:
Addison's disease: increased pigmentation of skin, weight loss, muscle wasting, tiredness, low blood pressure, diarrhoea and vomiting, confusion, collapse with dehydration	***/**	A33. Red flags of other endocrine diseases

Notes

– An altered mental state may be the result of a psychiatric condition, such as psychosis or extreme depression, or may have a physical (organic) basis. There are many organic causes of a confusional state, including drug intoxication, brain damage, epilepsy, high fever and a whole range of serious medical illnesses (e.g. pneumonia, diabetes, urinary infection). Confusion is more likely to develop in elderly people and young children in response to medical illness than is the case in older children and younger adults.

– There are two priorities to consider if a person is experiencing an altered mental state. First, that their behaviour may lead to harm to themselves or those around them; and second, that the underlying medical condition may merit urgent attention.

First-aid measures for altered mental state

- Call for medical assistance.
- Ensure the patient is kept calm. If you are concerned about the patient's immediate safety or that of those around them, it may be appropriate to call the police. Do not put yourself at risk.
- If you have reason to suspect hypoglycaemia (confusion/agitation in a known diabetic), then, as long as it is safe for you to do so, administer a glucose drink or sugar.
- If there is any deterioration in consciousness, ensure the patient is kept safe and place in the recovery position with the airway open.
- Continue to check airway, breathing and circulation (ABC). If breathing, keep in the recovery position. If not breathing, call emergency services and be prepared to perform cardiopulmonary resuscitation (CPR).

TABLE C9 Red flags of diseases of the skin

Symptoms suggestive of:	Priority	For more detail and definitions go to:
Bruising and non-blanching rash, with severe headache and fever: suggests meningococcal meningitis	***	A23. Red flags of headache
Bruising and non-blanching rash with severe malaise: suggests meningococcal septicaemia	***	A11. Red flags of diseases of the blood vessels
Purpura or bruising rash (non-blanching): suggests a bleeding disorder or vasculitis. Refer urgently if rapidly worsening	***/**	A41. Red flags of diseases of the skin

TABLE C9 Continued

Symptoms suggestive of:	Priority	For more detail and definitions go to:
Progressive swelling of the soft tissues of the face and neck (angio-oedema) and/or urticaria (nettle rash): refer urgently if there are any features of respiratory distress (itchy throat/wheeze)	***	A41. Red flags of diseases of the skin
Large areas of redness affecting most (>90%) of the body surface (erythroderma): refer because of the risk of dehydration and loss of essential salts	***/**	A41. Red flags of diseases of the skin
Early shingles: intense, one-sided pain, with overlying rash of crops of fluid-filled reddened and crusting blisters. The pain may precede the rash by 1–2 days. Refer for early consideration of antiviral treatment	**	A25. Red flags of diseases of the spinal cord and peripheral nerves

Notes

Most skin diseases do not merit emergency referral. There are only a few situations in which emergency referral might be considered for a skin condition:

– A purpuric rash (non-blanching violaceous macules) in the presence of extreme malaise or headache or vomiting (suggest meningococcal septicaemia).

– A blistering rash on one side of the body, especially in an elderly person (suggests shingles, which can benefit from urgent treatment with antiviral drugs), and especially if affecting the region of the ophthalmic distribution of the trigeminal nerve, as ocular involvement can threaten sight.

– Angio-oedema: acute swelling of tissues, with urticaria and breathlessness (features of anaphylactic shock).

– Erythroderma: generalised inflammation of the skin wherein most of the skin surface is affected (due to eczema, psoriasis, sun exposure or drug reactions). There is a risk of circulatory collapse from poor fluid control. Refer urgently if any signs of shock are present.

First-aid measures for meningococcal septicaemia

● Call for medical assistance.
● Ensure the patient is kept still and calm.
● If there is any deterioration in consciousness, ensure the patient is kept safe and is placed in the recovery position with the airway open.
● Continue to check airway, breathing and circulation (ABC). If breathing, keep in the recovery position. If not breathing, call emergency services and be prepared to perform cardiopulmonary resuscitation (CPR).

First-aid measure for shingles

● Arrange medical assistance; the important issue is to take medication as soon as possible.

First-aid measures for anaphylactic shock and erythroderma

● See above under 'blood loss and shock' (**C3**) and 'acute difficulty in breathing' (**C4**).

TABLE C10 Red flags of headache

Symptoms suggestive of:	Priority	For more detail and definitions go to:
Subarachnoid haemorrhage: a sudden very severe headache that comes on out of the blue. The patient needs to lie down and may vomit. There may be neck stiffness (reluctance to move the head) and dislike of bright light	***	A23. Red flags of headache
Rapid increase in intracranial pressure (intracranial haemorrhage): headache followed by a rapid deterioration of consciousness leading to coma. Irregular breathing patterns and pinpoint pupils are a very serious sign. May be spontaneous or may result from a head injury	***	A21. Red flags of raised intracranial pressure A22. Red flags of brain haemorrhage, stroke and brain tumour
Severe headache that develops over the course of a few hours to days, with fever, and together with either vomiting or neck stiffness: possible acute meningitis or encephalitis	***	A23. Red flags of headache
Meningococcal septicaemia: acute onset of purpuric rash, possibly accompanied by headache, vomiting and fever	***	A11. Red flags of diseases of the blood vessels
Malignant hypertension: diastolic pressure >120 mmHg, with symptoms: including recently worsening headaches, blurred vision and chest pain	***/**	A12. Red flags of hypertension
Pre-eclampsia/HELLP syndromes: headache, abdominal pain, visual disturbance, nausea and vomiting, and oedema (in middle to late pregnancy)	***	A37. Red flags of pregnancy
Temporal arteritis: severe one-sided headache over the temple occurring for the first time in an elderly person or in someone with polymyalgia rheumatica. Blurring or loss of sight are very serious signs	***/**	A23. Red flags of headache

Notes

– Headaches are common and are usually benign.

– In rare cases, headaches might signify a disorder of the brain, such as an infection, haemorrhage, thrombosis or a tumour. In all these situations there are characteristic features (see **A23**) which will help distinguish these headaches from benign headaches (i.e. tension headache and migraine).

– In only rare situations will a patient with a headache merit an emergency response. Emergency situations include brain haemorrhage, brain infection, malignant hypertension, arteritis and pre-eclampsia in pregnancy.

First-aid measures for serious headache

● Call for medical assistance.
● Ensure the patient is kept still and calm.
● If there is any deterioration in consciousness, ensure the patient is kept safe and place in the recovery position with the airway open.
● Continue to check airway, breathing and circulation (ABC). If breathing, keep in the recovery position. If not breathing, call emergency services and be prepared to perform cardiopulmonary resuscitation (CPR).

TABLE C11 Red flags of diseases of the eye

Symptoms suggestive of:	Priority	For more detail and definitions go to:
Painful, red and swollen eye and eyelids: the patient (often a child) is very unwell (orbital cellulitis)	★★★	A42. Red flags of diseases of the eye
A painful red eye: most causes need high-priority/ urgent treatment (e.g. corneal ulcer, uveitis, scleritis, foreign body lodged in the eye)	★★★/★★	A42. Red flags of diseases of the eye
Sudden onset of painless blurring or loss of sight in one or both eyes accompanied by one-sided headache in someone over 50 years old: suggestive of **temporal arteritis**. There is a high risk of further loss of sight or stroke. Refer for urgent treatment with corticosteroids	★★★	A42. Red flags of diseases of the eye
Sudden loss of sight in a painless eye: could be thrombosis of the retinal artery, damage to the optic nerve or multiple sclerosis. Refer as soon as possible, in case it is the treatable retinal tear	★★★	A42. Red flags of diseases of the eye
Blurred vision in malignant hypertension: diastolic pressure >120 mmHg with symptoms, including recently worsening headaches, blurred vision and chest pain	★★★/★★	A12. Red flags of hypertension
Blurred vision in pre-eclampsia/HELLP syndromes: headache, abdominal pain, visual disturbance, nausea and vomiting, and oedema (in middle to late pregnancy)	★★★	A37. Red flags of pregnancy
Ophthalmic shingles: intense, one-sided pain over the forehead and eye, with an overlying rash of crops of fluid-filled reddened and crusting blisters. The pain may precede the rash by 1–2 days. Refer for early consideration for antiviral treatment, especially in the elderly	★★	A25. Red flags of diseases of the spinal cord and peripheral nerves
Discharge from the eyes in the newborn: could signify gonococcal or chlamydial infection (contracted during delivery), both of which pose a risk for the baby	★★	A42. Red flags of diseases of the eye

TABLE C11 Continued

Symptoms suggestive of:	Priority	For more detail and definitions go to:
Inability to close the eye: (in thyroid eye disease and also in Bell's palsy). Risk of damage to the conjunctiva and cornea. Keep the affected eye shut with a pad held in place with medical tape until medical advice has been sought	**	A42. Red flags of diseases of the eye
Foreign body in the eye: if not possible to remove, gently keep the lid closed by means of a pad and medical tape and arrange urgent assessment at the nearest eye emergency department	**	A42. Red flags of diseases of the eye

Notes

– The eyes are very vulnerable to infection and injury, and in some cases disease merits urgent referral for early treatment to prevent long-term damage.

– Visual disturbance may also be a red flag of disturbances of neurological function, such as stroke, malignant hypertension and toxaemia of pregnancy.

First-aid measures for eye problems

● Call for medical assistance or arrange for the patient to visit an eye casualty department.
● If you suspect a retinal tear, keep the patient calm and still.
● If you suspect a foreign body or a corneal ulcer, or if the eye cannot close, gently close the eyelid by means of a small pad and medical tape.

TABLE C12 Red flags of thromboembolism in the limbs

Symptoms suggestive of:	Priority	For more detail and definitions go to:
Limb infarction (suddenly extremely pale, painful, mottled and cold limb): results from a clot in a major artery. The life of the limb is threatened	***	A11. Red flags of diseases of the blood vessels
Features of a deep venous thrombosis (DVT): a hot swollen tender calf, can be accompanied by fever and malaise. There is an increased risk after air travel and surgery, and in pregnancy, cancer and if on oral contraceptive pill	**	A11. Red flags of diseases of the blood vessels
Thromboembolism in pregnancy: pain in the calf or breathlessness, with chest pain, or blood in the sputum in pregnancy or the puerperium. These symptoms and signs are serious at all times, but are more likely to develop in pregnancy and the puerperium, as there is an increased tendency for the blood to form clots at these times	***	A37. Red flags of pregnancy

Notes

– The development of a blood clot in an artery is a serious condition, as the blood supply to the tissue supplied by the blocked artery will be cut off, and thus immediately threaten the life of that tissue. The red flags of infarction of the brain (stroke), coronary arteries (heart attack), lung (pulmonary embolism) and bowel (leading to acute abdomen and shock) have been described earlier under 'loss of consciousness' (**C7**), 'chest pain' (**C5**) and 'acute abdominal pain' (**C1**). Infarction of a limb is one other situation in which thrombosis of an artery merits an emergency response.

– The development of a blood clot in a vein is serious, not because the tissues are greatly threatened, but because a part of the blood clot may break off and travel to lodge in the pulmonary circulation. This event can cause a life-threatening pulmonary embolism.

First-aid measures for infarction of a limb or deep vein thrombosis

● Call for medical assistance.
● Keep the patient calm and still, and discourage use of the affected limb.

CHAPTER 5

COMMUNICATING WITH MEDICAL PRACTITIONERS

It is good both for patient care and also for interprofessional relationships that complementary medical practitioners maintain contact with the conventional medical practitioners who are involved in the ongoing healthcare of their patients. One important reason for complementary therapists to communicate with conventional doctors is to refer patients who demonstrate red flag conditions, so that the patient can access relevant medical advice and treatment. If the communication is made in a way which is both valid in terms of patient care and respectful of the professional to whom it is directed then it can only serve to improve relationships between complementary and conventional medical practitioners. In this way it can serve to promote the ideals of integrated health care.

CHOICE OF METHOD OF COMMUNICATION

There are three methods by which a complementary medical practitioner might choose to communicate with a conventional medical doctor about a patient. By far the most commonly used and convenient method is to allow the patient to do the communicating by making an appointment with their doctor. Alternatively the practitioner can telephone the practice or hospital to speak to the patient's health care professional in person. The most formal approach is to write a letter. These three approaches will be considered in turn.

USING THE PATIENT AS THE COMMUNICATOR

The most usual clinical situation in which it may help for the patient to communicate something about a complementary health consultation with their doctor is when a non-urgent red flag has been identified. An example of this is the situation when an elderly patient mentions they have been more thirsty than usual for the past 3 months and have been passing large amounts of urine (red flag of type 2 diabetes). In this situation the patient needs to be advised to make an appointment with their doctor so that the possibility of serious disease can be excluded or confirmed.

At the appointment, the patient can then explain to the doctor that their practitioner is concerned about their symptoms and that, for example, there is a possibility of diabetes. In many such situations, a letter is not necessary.

As long it is clear to the therapist that the necessary information can be communicated effectively by the patient, this may be the most empowering option for them.

SPEAKING TO THE DOCTOR IN PERSON

Speaking to the doctor in person is the preferred mode of communication either if a patient needs to be referred urgently or if there is a matter of some complexity which needs to be discussed. Most doctors would be very happy to discuss a problem concerning a patient over the telephone (for example 'Mrs Jones, who lives alone, seems to have been getting progressively more confused. Are you aware of this?'). Whenever possible, it is important to ensure that the patient is told in advance what is going to be said to ensure that there is no breach of confidentiality.

It is normal in UK general practice to have systems in place where doctors make telephone consultations on request, usually at a particular time of the day. However, in a situation of high urgency, the duty doctor may be contacted straight away. The practice receptionist is trained to discern which calls merit urgent handling. If the call is after office hours, then it will be transferred to an 'on-call' doctor when the practice telephone number is called. It is important to bear in mind that the doctor who is contacted may not know the patient, or have any access to details about them, although in office hours the doctor should have electronic access to patient records.

COMMUNICATING BY LETTER

The letter is an appropriate method of referring complex patients and also of communicating clinical information about a patient in a non-urgent situation. A letter is not appropriate if information or advice is required, as the process of writing a reply is inconvenient for a busy doctor, and delays may occur if a letter has then to be typed and posted. If a problem needs to be discussed, such as Mrs Jones' confusion, then the telephone is the best medium.

A letter is most useful when it either precedes or accompanies a patient who has made an appointment with the doctor. The letter can then communicate the additional information which it may be important to impart.

THE STRUCTURE AND CONTENT OF THE COMMUNICATION

Whenever a referral is made, clear and succinct information needs to be imparted to the medical practitioner. Whether by the spoken word or by letter, this is best done in a structured way, and with the information offered in an order which is familiar to the doctor. If it is necessary to communicate by telephone, it is worthwhile for the complementary medical practitioner to prepare the information to be communicated in a systematic way before making contact.

A list of the categories of information summarised below can be a useful aide-mémoire to ensure no important details are omitted from either a telephone call or in the writing of a letter. Referring to the list will also help ensure that all the necessary information is given in a logical order. General practitioners and hospital doctors tend to be overburdened with paperwork, and so it is important that telephone calls and referral letters offer information in brief and accessible format. It helps to keep written information in terse bulleted statements, and to confine a letter to less than one page in length.

In the UK, there is legislation designed to protect the rights of patients so that sensitive information about them is stored in a safe way. The Data Protection Act 1998 requires practitioners to register if they intend to keep electronic records of sensitive information about patients. This is not necessary if electronic copies of the letters are deleted once they have been printed out, in which case paper copies can be kept for the patient records.

INFORMATION TO INCLUDE WHEN COMMUNICATING ABOUT A PATIENT TO A MEDICAL PRACTITIONER

Patient identifiers

Give full name, date of birth and address. All three of these are required for medical records.

Brief summary of reason for referral

In one sentence: something like: 'I'd be grateful if you could assess this 28-year-old man who tells me he has had three episodes of nocturnal bed wetting.'

More detailed history of main complaint

A brief synopsis of the key events in the history of the main complaint, including:

Symptoms
Describe the symptoms as described by the patient.

Signs
Then describe any findings (including relevant negatives like 'blood pressure was normal') on clinical examination.

Drug history
Summarise the medication the patient is currently taking (including contraceptives and non-prescribed medication such as indigestion remedies).

Social history
List any relevant lifestyle factors such as smoking, alcohol use and occupational factors which might have impacted on the current condition.

Summarise what is wanted of the medical practitioner

For example: 'I am concerned that this man might be experiencing nocturnal seizures, and would value your opinion on whether he needs further investigations.'

If appropriate, take the opportunity to describe how you have been treating with complementary medicine

A referral is a good opportunity to explain more about what complementary medicine involves. It is probably best not to use too much professional jargon in a referral situation, but a couple of sentences on why the patient is having complementary therapy and how they are benefiting can do no harm.

IMPORTANT ADDITIONAL POINTS WHICH APPLY TO LETTERS

The important points to follow when structuring letters are as follows:

Headed notepaper (see Figure 5.1)

Headed notepaper should include the name of the practitioner, professional title and qualifications, address, telephone numbers, fax number, e-mail address and Web site address.

Date

The date of the letter is essential.

Choice of language

It will help with all communications if the practitioner aims to match the medical use of professional language as much as possible, and to avoid using

Dr George Jackson
The Springs Surgery
Reading RG2 3DD

Jane Goodson RGN LicAc MBAcC
Traditional Chinese Medicine
The Willows Clinic
Reading RG1 IOU
Tel: 01189 222222, Fax: 01189 222223
jgoodson@acupuncture.com

12 April 2010

Dear Doctor Jackson

Re: ... include all patient identifiers here (i.e. name, address and date of birth) ....

Contents of letter ....
....

Yours sincerely
Jane Goodson

Figure 5.1 A guide to the basic information required on a professionally headed letter. (From CTG Table 6.3c1.)

complementary medical terminology which may be misinterpreted or dismissed as meaningless.

Confidentiality

Although letters between conventional health professionals are often written and sent without the express permission of the patient, it is advisable whenever possible to ensure that the patient is happy for you to be writing to another professional about them, even if they have been originally referred to you by that professional. A helpful hint is to always write a letter which you would be prepared for the patient to read. There should be very few situations in which it is legally advisable give information to the doctor without the patient knowing about it.

SAMPLE LETTER FOR REFERRING PATIENTS TO MEDICAL PRACTITIONERS

The use of standard letter format as indicated in Figure 5.2 is advised for the referral of patients who merit the opinion or treatment of a conventional medical

---

Dear Dr Jackson

I would be grateful if you could see John Smith with regard to unexplained back pain and weight loss.

I am treating him with acupuncture, but in view of his symptoms I believe he needs further investigations.

History
2 years of increasing low back pain, which first came on while digging.
In recent months pain has been constant, and not responsive to simple painkillers.
5 weeks ago he booked an appointment with me for pain relief.
Loss of 3 kg over the past year.
Poor appetite.
Night sweats and exhaustion over the past 3 months.

Examination
Pale, thin, general muscle wasting.
Abdominal exam: no obvious organ enlargement.
Very tender over the body of L3 vertebra with associated muscle spasm.

Medication
Co-codamol 1–2 tablets up to 4 times a day.

Treatment plan
I intend to see Mr Smith on a weekly basis, My treatments will involve gentle stimulation of acupuncture points to boost the depleted energy, and the use of points local to L3 to minimise pain.

This treatment would be entirely complementary to any treatment you may decide that he requires.

Many thanks for your help.

Yours sincerely
Jane Goodson

Figure 5.2 Sample referral letter. (From CTG Table 6.3c-IV.)

practitioner. In such a letter, it is important to clearly describe the red flags which are of concern. A medical diagnosis is not required in such a letter as the red flags will usually speak for themselves.

In urgent situations, a hand-written letter is perfectly acceptable. Hand-written letters should be structured in exactly the same way as typed letters.

In all cases, letters should be on headed notepaper and contain the general information about the patient and the referrer as indicated in Figure 5.1.

The letter in Figure 5.2 indicates that the practitioner has questioned and examined the patient appropriately and has discerned a red flag situation, a condition in which there is bone pain and also unexplained weight loss. The red flags of concern are described at the beginning of the letter. The structured approach to listing information as described earlier in this chapter has been adhered to. The doctor who receives this letter will be in no doubt that the patient needs urgent investigation to exclude malignancy or some other serious chronic disease such as TB, and will recognise that the patient's situation has been handled safely and professionally by the therapist.

CHAPTER 6

RED FLAGS AND REFERRALS: ETHICAL POINTS

This final brief chapter is concerned with some of the ethical issues which specifically relate to the situation of a complementary therapist who is considering the management of patients' symptoms and how they relate to red flags of serious disease. As described earlier, these red flag guides do not constitute imperatives for referral, but instead indicate those situations in which a complementary therapist needs to stop to consider whether or not referral might be appropriate for their patient.

As long as a therapist can be demonstrated to have made a sensible evidence-based clinical decision about whether or not to refer, and to have considered the best possible interests for the patient and the wider community in that decision, then whatever the outcome for the patient, it is unlikely that the therapist can be accused of behaving either unprofessionally or unethically. For evidence like this to stand up in the case of an investigation, there need to be clear contemporaneous records of the clinical decision-making process.

THE IMPORTANCE OF CLEAR RECORDS

It is a cardinal rule of clinical practice that should an ethical dilemma arise in practice then clear documentation of all relevant issues in the case notes needs to be made at the time. In particular, details should be recorded concerning the treatment and its rationale, any advice given, what has been discussed with the patient and its date. A practitioner's records are always used in an investigation of possible professional misconduct. If the records can demonstrate that the practitioner was following good practice as defined by their professional body in their dealings with a patient who has subsequently suffered harm or who has made a complaint, then the practitioner is unlikely to be disciplined.

For example, a practitioner could ensure that a clear record was made of the fact she had suggested that a patient should consult her GP for investigations into post-menopausal bleeding. In particular, she could clarify that she described the possible serious causes of this symptom, and that only medical tests could exclude these causes. If the patient is in sound mind but resists seeking a medical opinion, this ideally should be recorded. If the patient later makes an official complaint that she had a delayed diagnosis of womb cancer because her therapist said 'she would cure her', the fact that a discussion about referral at an early stage in the disease was clearly recorded at the time will obviously stand in the practitioner's favour (should the complaint come before an investigating committee).

For this reason, it is essential for practitioners never to make alterations to clinical records at a later date, even if what is written down is accurate. If it is necessary to add extra information to earlier records, then it should be dated with the date of addition. Altered records which are not dated as such will be seen as compromised, and effectively falsified, by an investigating committee. It is important to note that even 'tidying' records by reproducing in better writing an exact copy of original records is enough to cast doubt on their authenticity.

IF IN DOUBT, SEEK ADVICE

If a practitioner has any uncertainties about a particular case in practice or if a complaint has been made about an aspect of treatment, it is wise for them to consult either the professional conduct officer of their professional body or their insurer before taking further action.

MAINTAINING CONFIDENTIALITY

All health care practitioners have a duty to keep all information concerning their patients, medical or otherwise, entirely confidential. Such information should only be released with the explicit consent of the patient. This also applies to any views formed about the patient during consultations. To this end, when communicating with a doctor about a shared patient, it is advisable for practitioners to inform the patient in advance about the content of the letter or conversation to ensure they have given full consent to the information which is about to be disclosed.

However, there are times when patient confidentiality needs to be breached. This should only be done when the practitioner is convinced it is in the best interests of the patient or of society at large. For example, there might be genuine concern that an elderly person is becoming too confused to look after themselves, whereas they insist they are managing perfectly well. In this instance, it could be appropriate to make a telephone call to the GP to check that the practice is aware of the home situation of the elderly person.

If it is decided that it is in the best interests of the patient or to the wider community to disclose information about a patient, then clear records should be made of how that decision was made. If a practitioner has any uncertainties about whether or not to disclose confidential information in a referral, then it is wisest to discuss the situation first, in confidence, with their professional body. It must be emphasised that disclosure without consent is a very serious matter, and unless there is a serious risk of injury or harm to the public, it can be very difficult to justify. For example, even suicide threats are not usually thought to be a serious enough reason to disclose unless the means suggested may impinge on other people, e.g. driving a car recklessly or jumping off a shopping centre roof. Therefore, if there is any uncertainty about whether disclosure would be appropriate, it is wisest once again for the practitioner to consult in confidence with the professional conduct officer of their professional body.

Further reading

Ali, N., 2005. Alarm bells in medicine. Blackwell, Oxford.

British Medical Association. British Medical Journal. Available at: http://www.bmj.com.

British Medical Association and the Royal Pharmacological Society of Great Britain, 2011. British national formulary 62. Available at: http://www.bnf.org.

Bull, P.D., 1996. Lecture notes on diseases of the ear, nose and throat. Blackwell Science, Oxford.

Collier, J., Longmore, M., Brinsden, M., 2006. Oxford handbook of clinical specialities. Oxford University Press, Oxford.

Ellis, H., Calne, R., Watson, C., 2006. Lecture notes: general surgery, eleventh ed. Blackwell, Oxford.

Graham-Brown, R., Burns, T., 1996. Lecture notes on dermatology. Blackwell Science, Oxford.

Gray, D., Toghill, P., 2001. An introduction to the symptoms and signs of clinical medicine. Arnold, London.

Greer, I., Cameron, I., Kitchener, H., Prentice, A., 2001. Mosby's color atlas and text of obstetrics and gynaecology. Mosby, Philadelphia.

Health and Safety Executive, 2011. Health and safety guidance on first aid. Available at: http://www.hse.gov.uk/firstaid/.

Health Protection Agency, 2011. List of notifiable diseases. Available at: http://www.hpa.org.uk/Topics/InfectiousDiseases/InfectionsAZ/NotificationsOfInfectiousDiseases/ListOfNotifiableDiseases/.

Hopcroft, K., Forte, V., 2003. Symptom sorter, third ed. Radcliffe, Oxford.

James, B., Chew, C., Bron, A., 1997. Lecture notes on ophthalmology. Blackwell Science, Oxford.

Kumar, P., Clark, M., 2005. Clinical medicine, sixth ed. Elsevier Saunders, Edinburgh.

Lissauer, T., Clayden, G., 1997. The illustrated textbook of paediatrics. Mosby, Philadelphia.

Llewellyn-Jones, D., 1999. Fundamentals of obstetrics and gynaecology, Ch. 12. Mosby, Philadelphia.

Longmore, M., Wilkinson, I., Turmezei, T., Cheung, C.K., 2008. Oxford handbook of clinical medicine. Oxford University Press, Oxford.

National Institute for Health and Clinical Excellence (NICE). Clinical guidelines. Available at: http://www.nice.org.uk.

Oxbridge Solutions Ltd. A general practice notebook. Available at: http://www.gpnotebook.co.uk.

Puri, B.K., 2000. Saunders pocket essentials of psychiatry, second ed. WB Saunders, Philadelphia.

Index

Page numbers ending in 'f' and 't' refer to
Figures and Tables respectively

Printed in the United States
By Bookmasters